Task Oriented Gait Training

Yang-Soo Lee

Task Oriented Gait Training

Springer

Yang-Soo Lee
School of Medicine
Kyungpook National University
Daegu, Korea (Republic of)

ISBN 978-981-97-3347-7 ISBN 978-981-97-3348-4 (eBook)
https://doi.org/10.1007/978-981-97-3348-4

This Springer imprint is published by the registered company Springer Nature Singapore Pte Ltd.
The registered company address is: 152 Beach Road, #21-01/04 Gateway East, Singapore 189721, Singapore

Preface

Safe, independent gait is a critical function of humans, serving as a highly valuable means of moving from one place to another and significantly contributing to our quality of life. Moreover, it stands as a vital predictor of institutionalization and long-term survival. With the aging of the population and a decrease in mortality from life-threatening diseases, the number of people facing gait disabilities is expected to rise rapidly. Consequently, maximizing gait recovery has become a top priority in healthcare services.

Therefore, gait training is an integral component of rehabilitation, with its effectiveness well-established. However, in many cases, the outcomes of gait training fall short of expectations.

For instance, while gait training for individuals with chronic stroke results in notable improvements in mobility and gait speed, the magnitude of these effects remains limited. Additionally, there are no significant improvements observed in daily or social activities.

In light of these challenges, this book aims to address the complexities and nuances of gait training, exploring strategies and approaches aimed at enhancing its effectiveness and ultimately improve the lives of those with gait disabilities.

Thus, it is imperative that we refine the strategies of gait training. Nowadays, there is a growing consensus regarding the use of a task-oriented approach in gait training, as recommended by many guidelines. However, there is limited information available on specific strategies, their timing, and their appropriateness for different individuals.

A sound training strategy should align with established knowledge, such as neuroplasticity, learned nonuse, and the dose-effect relationship. There is a substantial body of evidence supporting neuroplasticity in humans, including within the adult nervous system. This allows us to set ambitious goals for gait training, aiming for normal or near-normal gait.

Many patients with gait disabilities exhibit learned nonuse of affected body parts, which can interfere with optimal training outcomes. The forced use of affected parts can prevent learned nonuse and maximize training effects.

While the relationship is not entirely linear, increasing the amount of training improves the outcomes of gait training. However, increasing the training amount with one-on-one training can lead to an unacceptable increase in healthcare costs. Thus, it is essential to utilize not only one-on-one training but also other training strategies, such as group training and independent training. Gait training should be effective in improving gait function, but other characteristics of training are equally important. To be widely adopted, it should be easy to learn, easy to implement (both for healthcare providers and people with gait disabilities), and should not require expensive equipment.

Since improved gait function tends to deteriorate over time due to detraining effects and aging, gait training is a lifelong process. Regular exercise is essential to reduce the deterioration of gait function, with repeated gait training necessary in the event of a significant decline in gait function.

The primary focus of this book is to provide practical knowledge regarding task-oriented gait training based on well-established principles. The step-by-step, task-oriented gait training outlined in this book aligns with the principles of value-based healthcare and may contribute to universal healthcare coverage.

The contents of this book have been developed with valuable feedback and comments from my patients, for which I am sincerely grateful. I also extend my appreciation to my wife, Soonyoung Lee, and my children, Junghyun, Jungwoo, and Sanghyun, who have provided encouragement and patiently awaited the completion of this book over a considerable period of time.

Daegu, Republic of Korea Yang-Soo Lee

Acknowledgment

I am deeply grateful for the invaluable assistance I have received in the creation of this book in the form of the works of esteemed authors and their seminal publications, specifically, *Neurological Rehabilitation: Optimizing Motor Performance 2nd Edition* and *Stroke Rehabilitation: Guidelines for Exercise and Training to Optimize Motor Skill*, authored by Janet H. Carr MA EdD (Columbia) FACP and Roberta B. Shepherd MA EdD (Columbia) FACP, as well as *Motor Control: Translating Research into Clinical Practice*, written by Anne Shumway-Cook PT PhD FAPTA, Marjorie H. Woollacott, et al. These exceptional works have been instrumental in shaping my understanding and approach to task-oriented gait training, which forms the foundation of this book. Their contributions to the field of neurological rehabilitation have been a guiding light, and I am indebted to their scholarship and insights.

Contents

Part I Introduction

1 Overview 3
1.1 Importance of Independent Gait 3
1.2 Requirements of Independent Gait 3
1.3 Prognosis of Gait Training 3
1.4 Goals of Gait Training 4
1.4.1 Long-Term Goals 4
1.4.2 Short-Term Goals 4
1.5 Need for Better Gait Training 5
1.6 Summary 5
References 6

2 Anatomy and Physiology 7
2.1 Anatomy 7
2.1.1 Joints 7
2.1.2 Neuroanatomy 9
2.1.3 Muscles 10
2.2 Physiology 10
2.2.1 Mode of Muscle Contraction 10
2.2.2 Sensory System 11
2.2.3 Synergy 12
2.2.4 Cognition 12
2.2.5 Balance 13
2.2.6 Dual-Task Interference 14
2.3 Pathophysiology 14
2.3.1 Motor Learning 14
2.3.2 Neuroplasticity 14
2.3.3 Weakness 14
2.3.4 Paresis 14
2.3.5 Detraining 15
2.3.6 Regaining Function 15
2.3.7 Learned Nonuse 15
2.3.8 Increased Muscle Tone 15
2.4 Summary 16
References 16

3 Normal Gait ... 19
3.1 Definition of Gait ... 19
3.2 Requirements of Normal Gait ... 19
3.3 Energy Conservation ... 19
3.3.1 Conversion of Energy ... 19
3.3.2 Minimizing Movement of the Center of Mass ... 20
3.3.3 Optimization of Muscle Contraction ... 21
3.3.4 Energy Storage and Release ... 21
3.4 Adaptation to Need ... 21
3.5 Velocity of Gait ... 21
3.6 Toe Out ... 21
3.7 Stride Width ... 22
3.8 Gait Cycle ... 22
3.8.1 Division of the Gait Cycle ... 22
3.8.2 Initial Contact Phase ... 22
3.8.3 Loading Response Phase ... 23
3.8.4 Mid-Stance Phase ... 23
3.8.5 Terminal Stance Phase ... 24
3.8.6 Pre-Swing Phase ... 24
3.8.7 Initial Swing Phase ... 25
3.8.8 Mid-Swing Phase ... 25
3.8.9 Terminal Swing Phase ... 25
3.9 Summary ... 25
References ... 26

4 Abnormal Gait ... 27
4.1 Effects of Abnormal Gait ... 27
4.2 Evaluation of Abnormal Gait ... 27
4.3 Causes of Abnormal Gait ... 27
4.3.1 Weakness ... 27
4.3.2 Loss of Flexibility ... 28
4.3.3 Pain ... 29
4.3.4 Sensory Disorders ... 29
4.3.5 Balance Problems ... 30
4.4 Classification of Abnormal Gait by Gait Pattern (Kinematics) ... 30
4.4.1 Causes of Abnormal Gait Patterns ... 30
4.4.2 Abnormal Movement of the Trunk ... 30
4.4.3 Abnormal Movement of the Pelvis ... 31
4.4.4 Abnormal Movement of the Hip ... 31
4.4.5 Abnormal Movement of the Knee ... 32
4.4.6 Abnormal Movement of the Ankle ... 32
4.4.7 Abnormal Movement of the Subtalar Joint ... 33
4.4.8 Abnormal Movement of the Toes ... 33
4.5 Summary ... 33
References ... 33

Part II Evaluation

5 Assessment of Gait 37
5.1 Assessment of Participation 37
5.1.1 Self-Reported Measures 37
5.1.2 Ambulatory Monitoring 37
5.2 Qualitative Tests Using Single Items 37
5.3 Classification of Gait Function 37
5.4 Quantitative Assessment Using Single Items 38
5.4.1 Gait Velocity 38
5.4.2 Timed Up and Go Test 38
5.4.3 Step Length 38
5.4.4 Stride Length 39
5.4.5 Step Frequency/Cadence 39
5.4.6 Step Width 39
5.4.7 Endurance 39
5.5 Assessment Using Gait Pattern (Kinematics) 39
5.5.1 Observational Gait Analysis 39
5.5.2 Optoelectric Analysis System 39
5.5.3 Systems Using Motion Sensors 40
5.5.4 Smartphone Apps 40
5.6 Assessment Using Kinetics 40
5.7 Summary 40
References 40

6 Assessment of Muscle Strength 43
6.1 Overview of Muscle Strength Test 43
6.1.1 Importance of Muscle Strength 43
6.1.2 Purpose of Muscle Strength Test 43
6.1.3 Proper Test of Muscle Strength 43
6.1.4 Field Tests 43
6.2 Manual Muscle Test 44
6.2.1 Overview of the Manual Muscle Test 44
6.2.2 Grading of Muscle Strength 44
6.2.3 Limitations of the Manual Muscle Test 46
6.3 Tests Using Closed Kinetic Chain Muscle Contraction 46
6.3.1 Heel Lift 46
6.3.2 Sit-to-Stand Test 47
6.3.3 Bridging 48
6.3.4 Squat Using Both Lower Limbs 49
6.3.5 Squat Test Using One Lower Limb 50
6.4 Dynamometer 50
6.4.1 Overview 50
6.4.2 Handheld Dynamometer 50
6.4.3 Isokinetic Dynamometer 50
6.4.4 Traction Dynamometer 51
6.5 Force Plate 51
6.6 Sliding Tilt Table 51

6.7 Test of Individual Muscles 52
6.7.1 Spinal (Back) Extensor 52
6.7.2 Hip Internal Rotator 52
6.7.3 Hip Flexor 52
6.7.4 Hip Abductor 53
6.7.5 Knee Extensor 53
6.8 Assessment of Power 53
6.9 Summary 53
References 54

7 Assessment of Balance 57
7.1 Importance of Balance 57
7.2 Role of Balance Tests 57
7.3 Principle of Balance Tests 57
7.4 Safety 57
7.5 Subjective Perception of Balance 58
7.6 Assessment of Steady-State Balance 59
7.6.1 Sitting Balance 59
7.6.2 Standing Balance 59
7.7 Assessment of Proactive Balance 60
7.7.1 Sitting Balance 60
7.7.2 Standing Balance 60
7.8 Reactive Balance 63
7.8.1 Reactive Sitting Balance 63
7.8.2 Reactive Standing Balance 63
7.9 Balance Test Batteries 64
7.9.1 Berg Balance Scale 64
7.9.2 Balance Evaluation System Test 64
7.9.3 Community Balance and Mobility Scale 65
7.9.4 Fullerton Advanced Balance Scale 65
7.9.5 Performance-Oriented Mobility Assessment 65
7.10 Tests Using Force Plates 65
7.11 Summary 65
References 66

Part III Training

8 Principle of Gait Training 71
8.1 Safety 71
8.2 Active Role of the Patient 71
8.3 Forced Use 71
8.4 Progressive Training 72
8.5 Feedback 74
8.6 Declarative Learning 74
8.7 Specificity of Training 74
8.8 Intensity 74
8.8.1 Amount of Training 74
8.8.2 Difficulty of Tasks 75
8.9 Motivation 75

8.10 Variable Training 75
8.11 Detraining 75
8.12 Gait Training Cycles 75
8.13 Facilitate Engagement with the Exercise Program 76
8.14 Summary 76
References. 77

9 **Muscle Strengthening**. 79
9.1 Relationship Between Strength and Gait. 79
9.2 Mechanisms of Muscle Strengthening. 79
9.2.1 Lower Motor Neuron Lesions 79
9.2.2 Upper Motor Neuron Lesions 79
9.3 Principles of Muscle Strengthening. 79
9.3.1 Appropriate Amount of Resistance 79
9.3.2 Postural Stability 80
9.3.3 Training Specificity 80
9.3.4 Control of the Effect of Gravity. 80
9.3.5 Mode of Strength Training. 81
9.4 Facilitation of Muscle Contraction 81
9.4.1 Functional Electrical Stimulation 81
9.4.2 Weight-Bearing 81
9.4.3 Change of Joint Alignment 81
9.5 Strengthening with a Closed Kinetic Chain Exercise 81
9.5.1 Bridging. 81
9.5.2 Sit-to-Stand 82
9.5.3 Squat with Two Legs 85
9.5.4 Single-Leg (Mini) Squat 86
9.5.5 Heel Lift. 86
9.6 Exercise with Elastic Band 90
9.7 Exercise with a Sliding Tilt Table 91
9.7.1 Components of the Sliding Tilt Table 91
9.7.2 Characteristics of a Sliding Tilt Table 91
9.7.3 Advantages of a Sliding Tilt Table. 92
9.7.4 Setup of a Sliding Tilt Table Before Exercise 93
9.7.5 Training with One Lower Leg 93
9.7.6 Training with Both Lower Limbs 96
9.7.7 Heel Lift Using a Sliding Tilt Table. 97
9.8 Strengthening of Individual Muscles. 99
9.8.1 Back Extensors. 99
9.8.2 Hip Flexors. 99
9.8.3 Hip Extensors. 101
9.8.4 Hip Abductors 102
9.8.5 Hip Internal Rotators 103
9.8.6 Knee Extensor Strengthening 106
9.8.7 Ankle Dorsiflexor Strengthening. 107
9.8.8 Ankle Plantar Flexor Strengthening. 107
9.9 Power Training. 108
9.10 Summary 108
References. 109

10 Balance Training 111
10.1 Effectiveness of Balance Training 111
10.2 Principles of Balance Training 111
10.2.1 Safety 111
10.2.2 Anxiety of Falling 111
10.2.3 Reduce the Base of Support 111
10.2.4 Movement of the Center of Mass 112
10.2.5 Progressive Training 112
10.3 Sitting Balance Training 113
10.3.1 Head Control Training 113
10.3.2 Steady-State Balance Training 113
10.3.3 Proactive Balance Training 114
10.3.4 Reactive Balance Training 115
10.4 Standing Balance Training 115
10.4.1 Steady-State Balance Training 115
10.4.2 Proactive Balance Training 118
10.5 Balance Training with Equipment 125
10.6 Reactive Balance Training 126
10.7 Summary 126
References 126

11 Flexibility 129
11.1 Importance of Flexibility 129
11.2 Maintaining Flexibility 129
11.3 Principles of Stretching 129
11.3.1 Focused Stretching 129
11.3.2 Minimize Resistance to Stretching 129
11.3.3 Appropriate Amount of Stretching 129
11.3.4 Sustained Stretch 130
11.4 Methods of Stretching 130
11.4.1 Manual Stretching 130
11.4.2 Stretching with Orthosis 130
11.4.3 Serial Casting 130
11.4.4 Stretching in a Standing Posture 131
11.4.5 Stretching with a Machine 131
11.5 Summary 132
References 132

12 Task-Specific Gait Training 133
12.1 Definition of Task-Specific Gait Training 133
12.2 Level Ground (Overground) Gait Training 133
12.3 Gait Training with a Cane 133
12.4 Gait Training with Parallel Bars 133
12.5 Gait Training with a Treadmill 133
12.6 Body Weight-Supported Training 134
12.6.1 Body Weight-Supported Overground Training 134
12.6.2 Body Weight-Supported Treadmill Training 134
12.7 Gait Training with Functional Electrical Stimulation 134
12.8 Gait Training with Robots 134

12.9 Summary 134
References. 134

13 Task-Oriented Gait Training 137
13.1 Definition of Task-Oriented Gait Training. 137
13.2 Evidence of Effectiveness of Task-Oriented Gait Training 137
13.3 Principles of Task-Oriented Gait Training 137
13.3.1 Strengthening Before Balance Training. 137
13.3.2 Maximize Function of the Affected Limb 137
13.3.3 Safety 138
13.3.4 Progressive Training 138
13.4 Sequence of Gait Training 138
13.4.1 Muscle Strengthening of Weight-Supporting Muscles 138
13.4.2 Training for Steady-State Standing Balance 138
13.4.3 Training for Proactive Standing Balance 139
13.4.4 The Reasons for Placing Overground Gait Training at the End. 140
13.4.5 Training People with Severe Ankle Plantar Flexor Weakness 140
13.5 Advantages of Step-by-Step Task-Oriented Gait Training . . 140
13.6 Summary 140
References. 141

14 Gait Training for People with Specific Diseases 143
14.1 Stroke 143
14.2 Traumatic Brain Injury. 143
14.3 Spinal Cord Injury 144
14.4 Parkinson's Disease 144
14.5 Cerebral Palsy 145
14.6 Knee Osteoarthritis 145
14.6.1 Hip Surgery 146
14.7 Elderly People with Gait Disability 147
14.8 Summary 148
References. 148

15 Abnormal Gait 151
15.1 Cautious Gait 151
15.2 Genu Recurvatum (Knee Hyperextension) 151
15.3 Poor Foot Clearance. 151
15.4 Gait with Foot Inversion 152
15.5 Circumduction Gait 152
15.6 Ataxic Gait. 153
15.7 Frontal Lobe Gait. 153
15.8 Summary 153
References. 153

16 Others . . . 155
16.1 Other Gait Training . . . 155
16.2 Training Using Dual Tasks . . . 156
16.3 Reactive Balance Training . . . 156
16.4 Training Going Up and Down Stairs . . . 157
16.5 Dizziness . . . 158
16.6 Sensory/Perception Test . . . 158
16.6.1 Hemispatial Neglect . . . 158
16.6.2 Proprioception . . . 158
16.7 Program to Maintain Function . . . 158
16.8 Walking Aids (Assistive Devices) . . . 159
16.8.1 Cane . . . 159
16.8.2 Stick . . . 160
16.8.3 Walker . . . 160
16.9 Orthoses . . . 160
16.9.1 Ankle-Foot Orthoses . . . 160
16.9.2 Knee Orthoses . . . 160
16.10 Summary . . . 160
References . . . 161

Part I

Introduction

1 Overview

1.1 Importance of Independent Gait

Gait, the repetitive and reciprocal movement in which the lower limbs are used to move from one place to another, stands as one of human beings' most crucial functions. Its significance can be observed from a variety of different viewpoints. Firstly, gait provides a convenient means for individuals to navigate various terrains, including ramps, stairs, uneven surfaces, and obstacles. Secondly, it serves as a valuable form of exercise and may even be the primary mode of physical activity for many, particularly those among the elderly population. Engaging in physical activity enhances physical function and is associated with a lower risk of developing conditions such as cognitive decline, dementia, colon and breast cancer, coronary heart disease, and type 2 diabetes (Gleeson et al. 2011). Reduced physical activity due to gait loss can result in various adverse consequences, including constipation, obesity, osteoporosis, and reduced cardiovascular fitness. Thirdly, many social activities require the ability to walk. Finally, dependent gait places a significant physical burden on caregivers. Therefore, regaining independent gait following disease or injury is closely linked to home discharge (Louie et al. 2022), and it is associated with longevity (Snijders et al. 2007; Bloem et al. 2000; Lear et al. 2017), improved health-related quality of life (Snijders et al. 2007), and enhanced community integration (Cohen et al. 2018).

1.2 Requirements of Independent Gait

Independent gait necessitates intact motor functions, sensory input, and perceptual cognitive abilities. Sufficient muscle strength is required for both supporting body weight and directing movement while the sensory function plays a crucial role in regaining the ability to walk efficiently. Finally, perceptual cognition is essential for identifying and avoiding potential risks, such as obstacles, uneven surfaces, irregularities, and moving vehicles.

1.3 Prognosis of Gait Training

Several factors, including age (Kollen et al. 2006), Barthel index score, sitting balance (EPOS study, Veerbeek et al. 2011), standing balance (Kollen et al. 2005), strength of the hemiplegic leg (EPOS study, Veerbeek et al. 2011), and sensation, are associated with the prognosis of gait training. However, predicting gait performance based on prognostic factors remains challenging for individuals with gait disabilities. That said, in some cases, individuals with severe motor impairment in the acute stage have shown significant gait recovery.

Y.-S. Lee, *Task Oriented Gait Training*, https://doi.org/10.1007/978-981-97-3348-4_1

1.4 Goals of Gait Training

1.4.1 Long-Term Goals

While task-oriented gait training is increasingly being recognized for its effectiveness, specific details regarding when and how to incorporate various tasks into gait training are still lacking. However, the long-term goals of one's gait training can provide insights into addressing these issues.

One of the most common long-term goals of gait training is community ambulation. Community ambulation requires stability, the ability to walk a sufficient distance, walking speed, as well as the ability to navigate various terrains, including curbs, slopes, stairs, and uneven surfaces. It also demands sufficient perceptual and cognitive functionality in order to manage obstacles and potential threats. Obstacles can be managed by stepping over them or walking around them, depending on one's perception of the obstacles. When facing potential threats, such as moving vehicles, cognitive function is necessary to adjust one's walking speed or path. However, community ambulation does not consider the presence of abnormal gait patterns or the use of walking aids. Abnormal gait patterns (e.g., circumduction, foot inversion, genu recurvatum, etc.) not only affect appearance but also increase energy consumption and the risk of tissue injury, but correcting abnormal gait patterns that have become established can be particularly challenging.

A more desirable goal for gait training is achieving normal gait, characterized by normal kinematics, kinetics, speed, and independence from walking aids. While individuals with severe motor impairment or sensory loss may have only a limited chance of regaining normal gait, establishing this long-term goal from the outset of training is absolutely crucial. In fact, focusing on community ambulation as the primary goal may actually miss the possibility of regaining normal gait and could lead to the adoption of abnormal gait patterns (including the use of walking aids), which may impede the restoration of normal gait. To achieve (near) normal gait, learned non-use of the affected lower limb must be prevented, and abnormal gait patterns must be avoided (Fig. 1.1).

1.4.2 Short-Term Goals

Regaining normal gait may require an extended period of training. Short-term goals play a crucial role in monitoring training progress and focus on improving underlying impairments, task capacities, and gait function. To ensure the effective tracking of progress, these goals should be both measurable and time-limited, with weekly goalposts set for inpatients and monthly goalposts for outpatients. For patients suffering from chronic gait impairments, it may be appropriate to establish longer intervals between short-term goals.

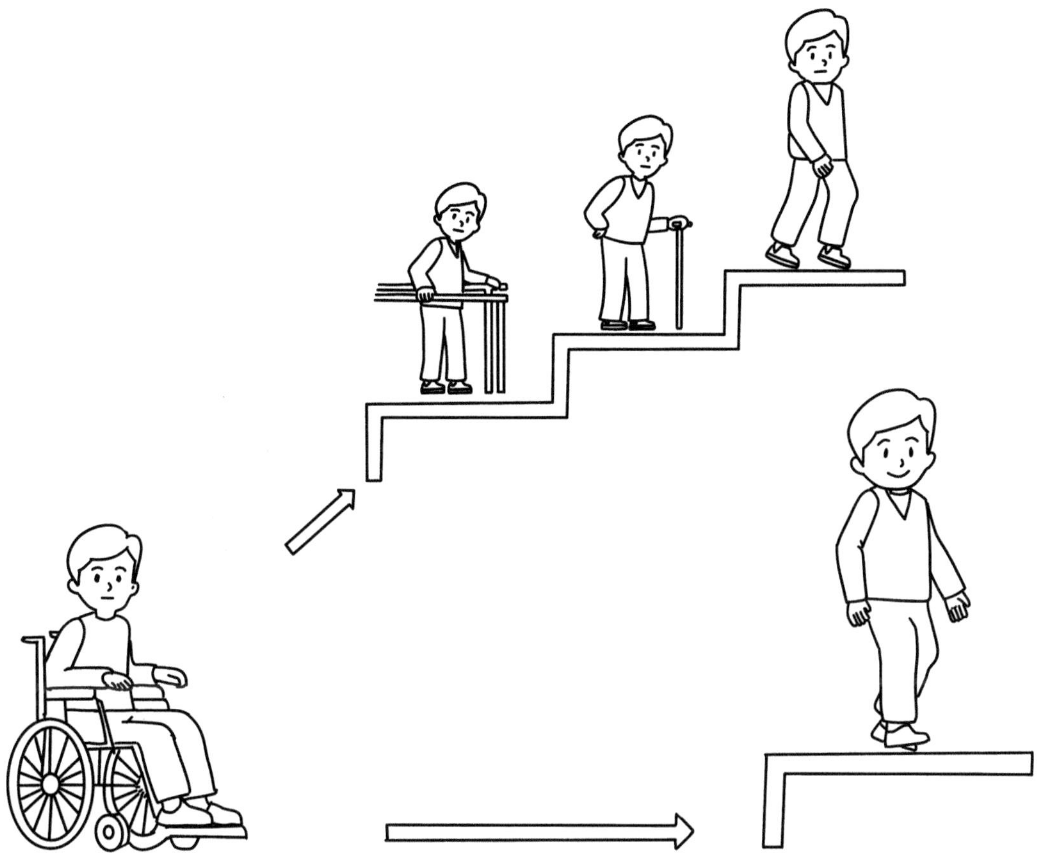

Fig. 1.1 Pursuing a normal walking pattern. To achieve normal gait, preventing the learned nonuse of the affected lower limb and avoiding abnormal gait patterns is essential

1.5 Need for Better Gait Training

Numerous research studies provide evidence of the effectiveness of task-oriented gait training (Allin et al. 2020; Bhatt et al. 2012, SC MC). However, in many cases, the outcomes of gait training have not been satisfactory. For instance, gait training for chronic stroke patients often results in a significant improvement in both mobility and gait speed, but its effects are still relatively modest (Green et al. 2002). Moreover, such training often results in no significant improvements in the patient's daily and social activities (Green et al. 2002). Thus, there is a pressing need to refine gait training strategies in order to achieve greater effects.

1.6 Summary

Gait serves as a fundamental method of moving from one place to another. Independent gait relies on motor function, sensory input, and perceptual cognitive abilities. It is also a vital contributor to overall health and a key aspect of social engagement.

As the prediction of gait training outcomes for individual cases is often vague and unreliable, it is all the more important to emphasize the strive for normal gait, especially in the initial stages of training.

References

Allin LJ, Brolinson PG, Beach BM, Kim S, Nussbaum MA, Roberto KA, Madigan ML. Perturbation-based balance training targeting both slip- and trip-induced falls among older adults: a randomized controlled trial. BMC Geriatr. 2020;20:205.

Bhatt T, Yang F, Pai YC. Learning to resist gait-slip falls: long-term retention in community-dwelling older adults. Arch Phys Med Rehabil. 2012;93(4):557–64.

Bloem BR, Gussekloo J, Lagaay AM, Remarque EJ, Haan J, Westendorp RG. Idiopathic senile gait disorders are signs of subclinical disease. J Am Geriatr Soc. 2000;48(9):1098–101.

Cohen JW, Ivanova TD, Brouwer B, Miller KJ, Bryant D, Garland SJ. Performance measures of strength, balance, and mobility predict quality of life and community reintegration after stroke? Arch Phys Med Rehabil. 2018;99(4):713–9.

Gleeson M, Bishop NC, Stensel DJ, Lindley MR, Mastana SS, Nimmo MA. The anti-inflammatory effects of exercise: mechanisms and implications for the prevention and treatment of disease. Nat Rev Immunol. 2011;11(9):607–15.

Green J, Forster A, Bogle S, Young J. Physiotherapy for patients with mobility problems more than 1 year after stroke: a randomised controlled trial. Lancet. 2002;359:199–203.

Kollen B, van de Port I, Lindeman E, Twisk J, Kwakkel G. Predicting improvement in gait after stroke: a longitudinal prospective study. Stroke. 2005;36(12):2676–80.

Kollen B, Kwakkel G, Lindeman E. Longitudinal robustness of variables predicting independent gait following severe middle cerebral artery stroke: a prospective cohort study. Clin Rehabil. 2006;20(3):262–8.

Lear SA, Hu W, Rangarajan S, Gasevic D, Leong D, Iqbal R, Casanova A, Swaminathan S, Anjana RM, Kumar R, Rosengren A, Wei L, Yang W, Chuangshi W, Huaxing L, Nair S, Diaz R, Swidon H, Gupta R, Mohammadifard N, Lopez-Jaramillo P, Oguz A, Zatonska K, Seron P, Avezum A, Poirier P, Teo K, Yusuf S. The effect of physical activity on mortality and cardiovascular disease in 130,000 people from 17 high-income, middle-income, and low-income countries: the PURE study. Lancet. 2017;390(10113):2643–54.

Louie DR, Simpson LA, Mortenson WB, Field TS, Yao J, Eng JJ. Prevalence of walking limitation after acute stroke and its impact on discharge to home. Phys Ther. 2022;102(1):pzab246.

Snijders AH, van de Warrenburg BP, Giladi N, Bloem BR. Neurological gait disorders in elderly people: clinical approach and classification. Lancet Neurol. 2007;6(1):63–74.

Veerbeek JM, Van Wegen EE, Harmeling-Van der Wel BC, Kwakkel G, EPOS Investigators. Is accurate prediction of gait in nonambulatory stroke patients possible within 72 h poststroke? The EPOS study. Neurorehabil Neural Repair. 2011;25(3):268–74.

2 Anatomy and Physiology

2.1 Anatomy

2.1.1 Joints

2.1.1.1 Hip Joint

The hip joint is formed at the meeting of the pelvic bone and femur head, and motion occurs in the sagittal, coronal, and transverse planes during gait. In the sagittal plane, motion occurs from 30° of flexion, from the mid-swing phase to the initial contact phase, to 10° of extension at the transition between the terminal stance phase and the pre-swing phase. In the coronal plane, 10° of adduction occurs by the end of the loading phase, and 5° of abduction occurs after toe-off. In the transverse plane, the total motion is 8°.

2.1.1.2 Knee Joint

The knee joint is formed at the meeting of the femur and tibia, and motion occurs in the sagittal, coronal, and transverse planes. Because even a small motion within the knee joint results in significant changes in either foot or body location, knee mobility and stability are major factors in gait function. Control of the knee joint is key to stance stability. Motion in the sagittal plane is large, at 60°, and shows two peaks of flexion during gait. The first small peak, at 20°, occurs at the transition between the loading phase and the mid-stance phase, and contributes to shock absorption. The second, larger, peak occurs during the initial swing and contributes to foot clearance. It is used for progression in the stance period and limb clearance, as well as advancement in the swing period. Motion in the coronal plane, at 8°, facilitates vertical balance over the limb during the single-limb support time. Motion in the transverse plane, at 6°, accommodates the changes in alignment due to the body's swing.

2.1.1.3 Talocrural Joint (Tibiotalar Joint)

Approximately 15° of plantar flexion and 10° of dorsiflexion occur at the talocrural joint during gait. To reduce the energy cost of gait, the movement of the center of mass should be minimized. The most important mechanism is the virtual lengthening of the lower extremity by ankle dorsiflexion at heel strike and ankle plantar flexion at pre-swing. Without ankle plantar flexion motion, the center of mass movement, and thus the energy cost of gait, increases. The axis of the joint is tilted 10° downward in the coronal plane with an inferior lateral end and 17° laterally directed in the transverse plane.

2.1.1.4 Subtalar Joint

The subtalar joint is an articulation between the talus and calcaneus (Fig. 2.1).

The most important function of the subtalar joint is the absorption of rotatory movement of the lower limb. When the human body experiences a toe-out movement while standing and walking, the axis of rotation of the talocrural joint is not congruent with the direction of progression. This problem must be solved to prevent

Y.-S. Lee, *Task Oriented Gait Training*, https://doi.org/10.1007/978-981-97-3348-4_2

tissue damage and gait instability. The subtalar joint has an obliquely oriented axis, allowing both inversion and eversion motion of the joint (Fig. 2.2).

Subtalar inversion results in the axis of the talus and midtarsal bones being incongruent, thus locking the movement of midtarsal joints and increasing foot stability. During terminal stance, the heel is lifted, requiring stability of the foot joint.

When the subtalar joint is everted, the talus and tibia internally rotate, causing the direction of progression and the axis of the ankle joint to be more congruent (Inman et al. 2005, ch1). This also contributes to shock absorption. Subtalar joint eversion also makes the talonavicular and calcaneocuboid joints parallel, allowing the foot to be more flexible.

2.1.1.5 Midtarsal Joints

There are many midtarsal joints, but the most important joints in relation to gait are the talonavicular joint and the calcaneocuboid joint. The movement of midtarsal joints in subtalar eversion contributes to shock absorption while subtalar inversion reduces the movement of midtarsal joints and increases foot stability.

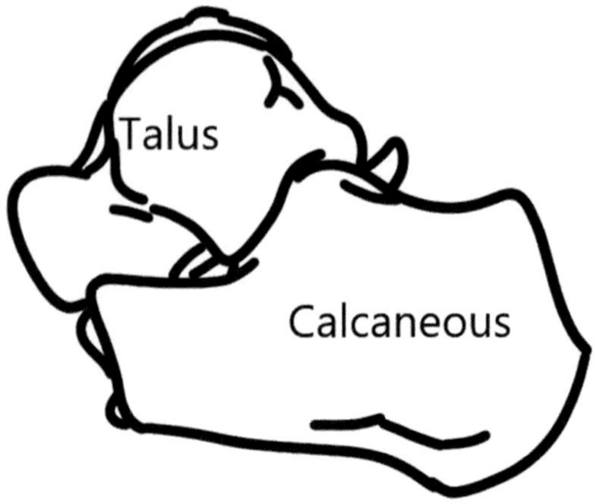

Fig. 2.1 Subtalar joint

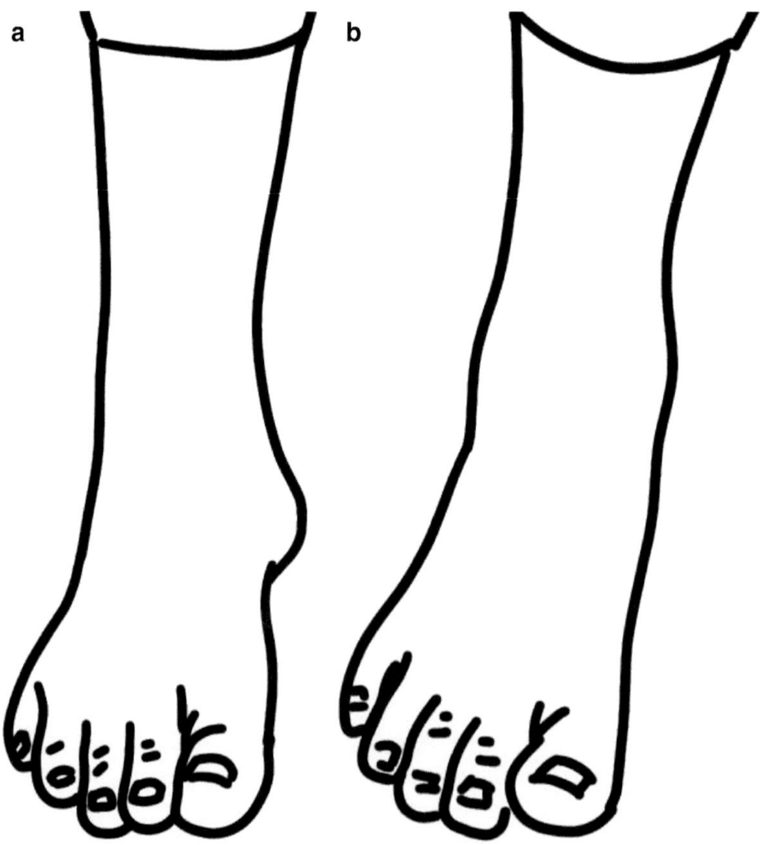

Fig. 2.2 Movement of the subtalar joint: (**a**) inversion; (**b**) eversion

2.1.1.6 Metatarsophalangeal Joints

The metatarsophalangeal joint normally allows for 55° of extension and enables the foot to roll over the metatarsal heads (forefoot rocker), creating the "toe break" of the shoe. The forefoot rocker is an important mechanism for facilitating the forward progression of the center of mass. In the midstance phase, the metatarsophalangeal joint remains in a neutral position. It progressively hyperextends from the terminal stance phase, reaching a maximal hyperextension of 55° just before toe-off. The plantar fascia attached to the proximal phalanx of the great toe supports the longitudinal arch and acts as a bow and string. With metatarsophalangeal joint extension, the plantar fascia tightens (via the Windlass effect), increasing foot stability. Limitation of motion in the metatarsophalangeal joints can cause pain and hinder the forward progression of the center of mass.

2.1.2 Neuroanatomy

2.1.2.1 Cerebral Cortex

Frontal Cortex

In humans, the motor cortex is more important for the function of locomotion than in other mammals (Pearson and Gordon 2000). Lesions in the motor cortex cause more severe paresis and gait disability in humans than in other mammals. Motor programs for gait modification on uneven surfaces and in response to upcoming threats are generated in the premotor cortex (Takakusaki 2013). Its activity is more pronounced in visually guided foot placement (Jensen et al. 2018; Petersen et al. 2012). The supplementary motor area contributes to postural control, and the planning and programming of locomotion.

Temporoparietal Cortex

The motor program is generated using the body schema, which is preserved in the temporoparietal cortex. This area of the brain is the most important in gait modification (Takakusaki 2013).

2.1.2.2 Basal Ganglia

The basal ganglia is involved in motor learning, the control of muscle tone and force, movement selection, and initiation.

2.1.2.3 Brainstem

The brainstem contributes to sensory-motor integration (Takakusaki 2013) and controls the descending motor pathways (reticulospinal tract and vestibulospinal tract). Lesions in the brainstem can cause paresis, motor ataxia, and postural instability.

2.1.2.4 Cerebellum

The cerebellum contributes to the correction of movement errors and the modulation of gait. The medial zone contributes to automatic gait control, and the lateral cerebellum contributes to novel context and visually guided modification (Takakusaki et al. 2008). Lesions in the cerebellum can cause severe ataxia.

2.1.2.5 Descending Motor Tract

Corticospinal Tract

The corticospinal tract is highly developed in humans, enabling skilled motions such as typing and writing. During gait, its activity is pronounced in visually guided foot placement (Jensen et al. 2018; Petersen et al. 2012). Lesions in the corticospinal tract cause paresis and loss of multi-joint coordination.

Reticulospinal Tract

The reticulospinal tract innervates both sides of the spinal cord and is crucial for regaining lost gait function in patients with severe lesions in the corticospinal tract. In stroke patients, the ipsilateral (nonaffected) hemisphere through the reticulospinal tract may contribute to regaining gait function (Jang et al. 2013).

2.1.2.6 Central Pattern Generator

The central pattern generator within the spinal cord generates rhythmic motion of the lower extremities. In animals, it has been found that gait-like motion can be produced with stimulation of the central pattern generator in the spinal cord. However, although the spinal pattern generator has been found to generate locomotor activity in experiments, gait production in humans has not been found to be possible without descending signals from higher centers (Pearson and Gordon 2000).

2.1.2.7 Motor Unit

The motor unit consists of the anterior horn cell (including axons), neuromuscular junctions, and innervated muscles. Lesions in the motor unit result in muscle weakness in lower motor neuron lesion.

2.1.3 Muscles

2.1.3.1 Paraspinal Muscles

Since paraspinal muscles are innervated by both hemispheres, they have the potential to recover after severe hemisphere damage.

2.1.3.2 Hip Flexor

The hip flexor is one of the major sources of energy that propels one's gait. Weakness of the hip flexor causes not only a compensatory gait pattern, such as hip circumduction, but also increased energy consumption.

2.1.3.3 Hip Abductors

There are three hip abductors: the gluteus maximus, gluteus medius, and tensor fascia lata. Weakness of hip abductors causes pelvic drop on the contralateral side or trunk tilt to the ipsilateral side in order to compensate for the weakness. Since the strength of hip abductors contributes to stability in the frontal plane, weakness increases fall risks in older adults (Krebs et al. 1998) and people with neurological pathology (Basford et al. 2003; Chou et al. 2003).

2.1.3.4 Tibialis Anterior

The tibialis anterior has the largest cross-sectional area among ankle dorsiflexors. Peak activity occurs at the initial contact phase. People with mild weakness of the ankle dorsiflexor demonstrate foot slap instead of foot drop.

2.1.3.5 Peroneal Muscles

For neutral ankle dorsiflexion, the activity of the tibialis anterior should be balanced with the activity of the peroneal muscles. If the activity of the peroneal muscles is inadequate, inversion of the subtalar joint occurs, increasing the risk of ankle inversion injury.

2.1.3.6 Calf Muscles

Calf muscle activity is the main energy source of gait, and the gastrocnemius and soleus muscles are the major calf muscles. Calf muscles are vital for maintaining balance while walking, and they play an important role in the recovery of balance. For the recovery of balance, the rate of force development is more important than muscle strength (Shumway-Cook et al. 2023a).

Soleus

The soleus is the largest muscle in the calf. This muscle contributes to body weight support and forward progression in gait (Neptune et al. 2001). Since it is attached to the medial part of the calcaneus, it is also a strong invertor.

Gastrocnemius

The gastrocnemius spans three joints—the knee joint, the tibiotalar joint, and the subtalar joint—and is attached to the lateral part of the calcaneus. Due to its attached point, it acts as an evertor. Contraction of the gastrocnemius leads to ankle plantar flexion and knee flexion. Knee flexion due to the contraction of the gastrocnemius facilitates hip flexion and initiates the swing (Neptune et al. 2001).

2.2 Physiology

2.2.1 Mode of Muscle Contraction

2.2.1.1 Open Kinetic Chain Muscle Contraction

In open kinetic chain muscle contraction, the distal parts of the body are moved. This muscle contraction utilizes the hip flexors, knee extensors, and ankle dorsiflexors in the swing period of the gait cycle to advance the lower limbs.

2.2.1.2 Closed Kinetic Chain Muscle Contraction

In closed kinetic chain muscle contraction, the head and trunk (rather than the distal parts of the body) experience movement through coordinated muscle contraction. In the stance period of the gait cycle, body weight support muscles—such as hip extensions, abductors, adductors, knee extensions, and ankle plantar flexors—use closed kinetic muscle contraction to support body weight. Closed kinetic chain muscle contraction minimizes shear forces across the joints and is task-specific in training body weight support muscles.

2.2.1.3 Concentric Muscle Contraction

In concentric muscle contraction, muscle length decreases during muscle contraction.

2.2.1.4 Eccentric Contraction

In eccentric contraction, muscle length increases during muscle contraction. Since eccentric contraction is used in gait to achieve shock absorption and decreased energy consumption, training with eccentric muscle contraction is extremely important. After experiencing a stroke, training with a focus on eccentric contraction may be more effective than focusing on concentric contraction in order to increase walking speed (Clark and Patten 2013).

2.2.1.5 Isometric Contraction

In isometric contraction, muscle length remains constant during muscle contraction. As exercises using isometric muscle contraction can decrease stress on the joint, this is often utilized in exercise for people with arthritis.

2.2.1.6 Co-contraction

Co-contraction of agonist muscles and antagonist muscles is an inefficient method of muscle contraction. It can be used by people with balance problems to compensate for poor balance as it increases joint stiffness and can help improve balance (Crenna 1998; Knutsson 1994). However, it increases energy consumption and leads to fatigue in people with poor aerobic capacity.

2.2.2 Sensory System

Sensory input is essential for learning, controlling, and adapting one's gait. In many sensory systems, the somatosensory, visual, and vestibular systems are more important than other sensory systems in gait.

2.2.2.1 Somatosensory System

Somatosensory input is very fast and is important for balance control and gait. In fact, its importance increases as tasks become more automatic. The main sources of somatosensory input are skin receptors, muscle spindles, and Golgi's tendon organs. In some situations, such as when walking across unstable surfaces or inclined surfaces, somatosensory information can become incorrect and require other sensory modalities for movement. Considering the consequences of somatosensory loss, it is an essential sensory modality for the sake of perception and movement.

Skin Receptors Sensory

Skin receptors provide input about the position and movement of the body. They also contribute to balance, especially reactive balance of the body.

Proprioception

Proprioception provides information about joint position (i.e., alignment of body segments), joint movement, and muscle contraction. It is extremely sensitive to postural disturbance and postural sway, and contributes to postural response. The sources of proprioception are muscle spindles, Golgi's tendon organs, and joint receptors. Sensory input from muscle spindles is the fastest sensory modality in the human body and allows for quick responses. For accurate sensing of joint motion, three sensory modalities—muscle spindles, skin sensory receptors, joint sensory receptors—are needed. If there is a problem with any one of them, proprioception decreases. Golgi's tendon organs provide information about the intensity of muscle contraction. A sufficiently stretched hip flexor at the end of the stance period excites the same muscle and inhibits the hip extensor, thus contributing to the transition from the stance to swing period.

2.2.2.2 Vision

Vision provides information about the environment, such as obstacles, moving vehicles, and the terrain of the path. But vision is also involved in proprioception. People perceive the position of their body using cues from the environment. One example is buildings, which are built vertically, as are flagpoles. Using this information, people can perceive the orientation of their body. As people can see the alignment of their body segments, this becomes very useful when other proprioception is severely impaired. However, these cues can be incorrect at times.

Movement is also perceived via visual flow information. As the body moves, the scenery changes. Still, it is possible to perform tasks with one's eyes closed. Thus, visual input is not essential for movement.

Unilateral spatial neglect (USN) is the inability to attend to information in unilateral space, and its severity can change depending on the task. For example, the ability to identify faces depends on the task. Although facial identification may be intact while sitting and standing, some people with stroke demonstrate impaired facial identification while walking. Since USN may be context-specific, testing while standing or walking may be necessary.

2.2.2.3 Vestibular Sensory

Vestibular sensory provides information about head orientation and motion. It is an absolute reference system and is especially important when visual and somatosensory systems provide conflicting input. Considering the difficulty that arises after the loss of vestibular sensory input, it is essential for movement. However, it is impossible to differentiate head motion from trunk motion using vestibular sensory input alone, so it must be used in conjuction with other sensory modalities.

2.2.2.4 Sensory Integration

In some instances, information from one sensory modality is incorrect and incongruent with other sensory modalities. In such cases, the central nervous system may neglect the sensory modality that seems incorrect and give more weight to other modalities that seem more accurate. However, this sensory integration is not always correct. For example, incorrect motion perception may occur when a car in another lane is moving.

2.2.2.5 Sensory Redundancy

Because there are three sensory modalities, the loss of one sensory modality can be compensated for by other modalities.

2.2.3 Synergy

Synergy in motor control refers to a stronger connection of several muscles than is typically found in the relationships between muscles. To simplify the control of movement, the nervous system utilizes synergy. It is often described in the following manner: "Muscle is to alphabet, synergy is to word, and action is to sentence" (Shumway-Cook et al. 2023b). For example, only 5–8 synergies are required for human gait (Chvatal and Ting 2013). Bernstein believed that synergies help solve the problem of degrees of freedom by causing muscles to work in unison. Usually, muscles belong to multiple synergies, and the activation of muscles is determined by the simultaneous activation of multiple synergies. It is essential to consider synergy when testing muscle strength and when attempting to strengthen muscles, as changes in joint angles can inhibit or facilitate muscle contraction.

2.2.4 Cognition

To achieve a normal gait, cognitive function is absolutely necessary. The first role of cognitive function is the strategic planning of the best route. If one cannot determine an appropriate route, achieving normal gait is impossible. Its second role is the acquisition of information regarding the external world as well as the adjustment of gait for safe movement. The third role of cognitive function is evaluating fall risk, which is determined by body function and environmental conditions. Underestimating risks can lead to falls and injuries (Snijders et al. 2007). The involvement of cognitive function in normal gait could explain the frequent falls seen in people with dementia (Snijders et al. 2007).

2.2.5 Balance

Balance control is a primary contributor to stable walking. Balance can be classified as steady-state balance, proactive balance, and reactive balance.

2.2.5.1 Steady-State Balance

The ability to maintain one's posture, such as while sitting or standing, was previously referred to as static balance. Although these postures may appear motionless, there is still very small motion present. Nowadays, it is referred to as steady-state balance. While sitting, motion can occur in the sagittal and coronal planes and is controlled by hip muscles, abdominal muscles, and back extensors. While standing, ankle motion is most important for steady-state balance.

2.2.5.2 Proactive Balance

Proactive balance is necessary for countering potentially destabilizing internal and external forces. This can be used interchangeably with anticipatory balance. Movement of one part of the body changes the location of the center of mass, and the body is moved without intention if there is no counteracting muscle contraction.

In addition, proactive balance may be conscious or subconscious. For instance, when people take hold of a previously unknown item, they first estimate its weight in order to prepare their body accordingly. This involves perception and cognition.

When people lift their right leg to take a step, counteracting muscle contractions are needed to prevent body perturbation. This action is usually performed subconsciously. Various nervous systems, including the supplementary motor cortex, basal ganglia, and cerebellum, are involved in proactive balance. Problems with proactive balance are common in people with gait disabilities. Proactive balance is required not only for gait initiation but also for complex walking tasks such as stepping over obstacles, changing directions, or adjusting walking velocity to avoid collisions. Almost all mobility tasks involve not only horizontal movement but also vertical movement of the center of mass (through lower extremity flexion and extension). Thus, tests and training should include components of vertical movement of the center of mass.

2.2.5.3 Reactive Balance

Reactive balance is necessary in order to recover balance following trips, slips, and unexpected perturbations. When loss of balance occurs, people use two kinds of strategies: the lower extremity strategy and the upper extremity strategy.

In the lower extremity strategy, somatosensory input is crucial because somatosensory input is faster than visual or vestibular input. If stepping is used to recover balance, visual input is also important for selecting a proper stepping location. Recovering balance from lateral movement of the center of mass involves lateral step and crossover step techniques, in which one leg crosses the midline of the body and the stance leg. In recovering from a trip using the lower extremity strategy, the critical muscles are the hip flexor of the swing leg and the ankle plantar flexors of the stance leg. In addition, the rate of torque development is more important than available strength (Chen 1993).

When utilizing the upper extremity strategy, known as reach and hold, visual input is more important than in the lower extremity strategy. This strategy requires information about the surrounding environment, such as distance and the stability of the base of support. Reactive balance responses in people with many neurological diseases are delayed and ineffective, significantly impacting functional independence. Thus, both testing and training of reactive balance are essential.

2.2.6 Dual-Task Interference

Dual-task interference refers to decreased performance when two tasks are conducted simultaneously, which can lead to falls and injuries. The tasks involved here can be classified as physical tasks and cognitive tasks. Physical tasks include sitting, standing, and walking, while cognitive tasks include calculations, memory tasks, and retrieval. The attentional requirement for dual-task performance depends on the individual's age, balance abilities, postural task, and sensory context.

2.3 Pathophysiology

2.3.1 Motor Learning

Motor learning, especially procedural learning, is classified under the umbrella of implicit memory, but it also involves explicit memory. When performing a sit-to-stand movement, many people with a gait disability place their foot anterior to the knee joint, which makes the sit-to-stand movement difficult. By teaching patients to place their foot posterior to the knee joint, leading to ankle dorsiflexion, it becomes possible to perform the sit-to-stand movement without the use of their hands. With the development of motor learning, the performance of tasks requires fewer attentional resources, allowing patients to perform other tasks simultaneously.

2.3.2 Neuroplasticity

Previously, it was believed that the adult central nervous system does not change. However, there has recently been ample evidence supporting neuroplasticity in the adult central nervous system. Neuroplasticity has a significant impact on the training of patients with gait problems. Even in cases of severe motor impairment, training can be conducted with the goal of recovering function (Nudo 2003). To induce neuroplasticity, repetition and motivation are crucial. Motivation increases when tasks are aligned with a person's desires, being functionally relevant and meaningful to them. While neuroplasticity can facilitate functional recovery, maladaptive neuroplasticity can lead to negative outcomes such as phantom pain and spasticity.

2.3.3 Weakness

People with muscle weakness lose the ability to generate adequate tone due to lesions in the motor unit (i.e., in the anterior horn cells, motor neuron axons, neuromuscular junctions, or muscles). Weakness can be improved through muscle hypertrophy and increased recruitment of anterior horn cells, both of which can be achieved via progressive resistance training.

2.3.4 Paresis

Paresis is caused by an upper motor neuron lesion, leading to insufficient supraspinal recruitment of motor neurons that innervate specific muscles. This problem can arise from issues related to the generation or conduction of a descending command to the motor unit. People with paresis experience a loss of the ability to generate adequate tone (i.e., weakness), an inability to contract muscles at the appropriate time (i.e., a timing problem), and an inability to contract muscles to an appropriate degree (i.e., a scaling problem). Due to these impairments, although muscle strength may remain the same, the function of individuals with upper motor neuron lesions (UMNL) is generally observed to be poorer than those with lower motor neuron lesions (LMNL). The scaling of muscle contraction is more challenging for individuals with paresis, making tasks requiring controlled eccentric contractions (such as descending stairs) more difficult than those requiring concentric contractions (such as ascending stairs). After a unilateral hemisphere lesion, the limbs on both sides of the body are affected, with the contralateral side being more severely affected and the ipsilateral side being less affected. On the less affected side, proximal muscles experience a stronger impact than do distal muscles.

2.3.5 Detraining

The effects of gait training can fade over time (Toulotte et al. 2006; Wolf et al. 2001). To maintain the positive effects of gait training, it is essential to aim for sustained functionality. As this is a lifelong process, the training should be both easy and cost-effective.

2.3.6 Regaining Function

Improvement occurs through synaptic plasticity and requires many repetitions.

2.3.6.1 Recovery

In the context of rehabilitation, recovery of function refers to regaining abilities through the use of the same kinetics and kinematics of the affected limb. Motor recovery refers not only to accomplishing tasks using the same end effectors but also to restoring the ability to perform a movement in the same manner typically seen in nondisabled individuals (Levin et al. 2009).

2.3.6.2 Compensation

In many cases, regaining function is achieved through compensation. Some researchers have shown that people with gait disability experience an increased walking speed with no change in their asymmetric gait after gait training, suggesting that improved function was due to compensation (Den Otter et al. 2006; Yu et al. 2015; Kwakkel and Wagenaar 2002). Although participants with chronic stroke walked faster after body-weight-supported treadmill training, the relative percentages of propulsion and positive work remained unchanged. These findings suggest that the increase in speed was likely due to compensatory strategies rather than through the recovery of normal kinetic symmetry (Combs et al. 2012). Regaining function through compensatory strategies can lead to negative clinical consequences such as an increased chance of musculoskeletal injury, increased energy cost and fatigue, overuse of the non-paretic leg, restricted walking activity, and an increased fall risk (Sánchez et al. 2015).

2.3.7 Learned Nonuse

Learned nonuse is a critical concept related to individuals with unilateral upper extremity dysfunction as it can interfere with the regaining of function in the affected upper extremity. In the lower extremity, both extremities are used during functional tasks such as transfers and gait. The term "learned misuse" may be more appropriately used to describe this phenomenon (Anjos et al. 2020). However, in terms of body parts, such as in the learned nonuse of the knee extensor, the concept of learned nonuse can be applied to the lower extremities. To prevent learned misuse of the lower extremities, hand usage needs to be minimized. Examples of hand usage include grasping, pulling, and placing one's hand on a table or wall. Grasping and pulling in sit-to-stand test not require forward body shifting using trunk flexion and lower extremity preparation, making it more likely to lead to learned nonuse of the trunk and the lower extremities. Placing one's hand on a table allows individuals to use their hand to support their body weight, potentially leading to learned nonuse. However, placing one's hand on a wall makes it impossible to support one's body weight, reducing the possibility of learned nonuse. Learned nonuse can occur not only with asymmetric impairments (e.g., hemiparesis, osteoarthritis, and total hip replacement) but also with symmetric impairments (e.g., lower extremity muscle weakness in the elderly). Learned nonuse may result in an asymmetric gait, impaired postural control, orthopedic problems (e.g., knee injury due to genu recurvatum), and spasticity. Targeted training for the involved body part may be necessary to prevent learned nonuse (Neptune et al. 2001). Various methods are utilized in targeted training, such as split-belt treadmills, sliding tilt tables, dummy prostheses, and adding weight to the non-paretic ankle.

2.3.8 Increased Muscle Tone

In the physiological range of motion, there is only minimal resistance to passive motion, allowing movement with only two fingers. If movement is difficult when using two fingers, this indicates increased muscle tone (Perry and Burnfield 2010, pp. 165–174). Increased muscle tone is caused by upper motor neuron lesions and presents as rigidity, spasticity, and spastic dystonia. Among these causes, spastic dystonia is relatively underexplored (Lumsden 2023). It refers to involuntary tonic muscle contractions in upper motor neuron lesions (Lumsden 2023). Spastic dystonia might also be more frequent than spasticity in individuals with stroke (Trompetto et al. 2019).

2.4 Summary

Because even a small motion of the knee joint results in significant changes in either foot or body location, knee mobility and stability are major factors in gait function. Control of the knee joint is key to stance stability.

To reduce the energy cost of gait, the movement of the center of mass should be minimized. The most important mechanism in this minimizing of movement is the virtual lengthening of the lower extremity by ankle dorsiflexion at heel strike and ankle plantar flexion at pre-swing.

The subtalar joint has an obliquely oriented axis, allowing inversion and eversion motions of the joint. When the subtalar joint is everted, the talus and tibia internally rotate, causing the direction of progression and the axis of the ankle joint to be more congruent.

The spinal pattern generator can generate locomotor activity in experimental animals, but it cannot produce gait without descending signals from higher centers in humans.

Balance control is a primary contributor to stable walking. Balance can be classified into three categories: steady-state balance, proactive balance, and reactive balance.

The effects of gait training can fade over time, so in order to maintain the positive effects of gait training, training that aims to sustain function is essential.

References

Anjos SD, Morris D, Taub E. Constraint-induced movement therapy for lower extremity function: describing the LE-CIMT protocol. Phys Ther. 2020;100(4):698–707.

Basford JR, Chou LS, Kaufman KR, Brey RH, Walker A, Malec JF, Moessner AM, Brown AW. An assessment of gait and balance deficits after traumatic brain injury. Arch Phys Med Rehabil. 2003;84(3):343–9.

Chen HC. Factors underlying balance restoration after tripping: biomechanical model analysis (Doctoral dissertation). University of Michigan; 1993.

Chou LS, Kaufman KR, Hahn ME, Brey RH. Medio-lateral motion of the center of mass during obstacle crossing distinguishes elderly individuals with imbalance. Gait Posture. 2003;18(3):125–33.

Chvatal SA, Ting LH. Common muscle synergies for balance and walking. Front Comput Neurosci. 2013;7:48.

Clark DJ, Patten C. Eccentric versus concentric resistance training to enhance neuromuscular activation and walking speed following stroke. Neurorehabil Neural Repair. 2013;27(4):335–44.

Combs SA, Dugan EL, Ozimek EN, Curtis AB. Effects of body-weight supported treadmill training on kinetic symmetry in persons with chronic stroke. Clin Biomech (Bristol, Avon). 2012;27(9):887–92.

Crenna P. Spasticity and 'spastic' gait in children with cerebral palsy. Neurosci Biobehav Rev. 1998;22(4):571–8.

Den Otter AR, Geurts ACH, Mulder T, Duysens J. Gait recovery is not associated with changes in the temporal patterning of muscle activity during treadmill walking in patients with post-stroke hemiparesis. Clin Neurophysiol. 2006;117(1):4–15.

Inman VT, Ralston HJ, Todd F. Human locomotion. In: Rose J, Gamble JG, editors. Human walking. 3rd ed. Philadelphia: Lippincott Williams & Wilkins; 2005. p. 1–18.

Jang SH, Chang CH, Lee J, Kim CS, Seo JP, Yeo SS. Functional role of the corticoreticular pathway in chronic stroke patients. Stroke. 2013;44(4):1099–104.

Jensen P, Jensen NJ, Terkildsen CU, Choi JT, Nielsen JB, Geertsen SS. Increased central common drive to ankle plantar flexor and dorsiflexor muscles during visually guided gait. Physiol Rep. 2018;6(3):e13598.

Knutsson E. Can gait analysis improve gait training in stroke patients. Scand J Rehabil Med Suppl. 1994;30:73–80.

Krebs DE, Jette AM, Assmann SF. Moderate exercise improves gait stability in disabled elders. Arch Phys Med Rehabil. 1998;79(12):1489–95.

Kwakkel G, Wagenaar RC. Effect of duration of upper- and lower-extremity rehabilitation sessions and walking speed on recovery of interlimb coordination in hemiplegic gait. Phys Ther. 2002;82(5):432–48.

Levin MF, Kleim JA, Wolf SL. What do motor "recovery" and "compensation" mean in patients following stroke? Neurorehabil Neural Repair. 2009;23(4):313–9.

Lumsden DE. Spastic dystonia: still a valid term. Dev Med Child Neurol. 2023;00:1–8.

Neptune RR, Kautz SA, Zajac FE. Contributions of the individual ankle plantar flexors to support, forward progression and swing initiation during walking. J Biomech. 2001;34(11):1387–98.

Nudo RJ. Adaptive plasticity in motor cortex: implications for rehabilitation after brain injury. J Rehabil Med. 2003;41:7–10.

Pearson K, Gordon J. Locomotion. In: Kandel ER, Schwartz JH, Jessell TM, editors. Principles of neural science. 4th ed. New York: McGraw-Hill; 2000. p. 737–55.

Perry J, Burnfield J. Pathological mechanisms (ch10). In: Gait analysis: normal and pathological function. 2nd ed. Thorofare: Slack Incorporated; 2010. p. 165–74.

Petersen TH, Willerslev-Olsen M, Conway BA, Nielsen JB. The motor cortex drives the muscles during walking in human subjects. J Physiol. 2012;590(10):2443–52.

Sánchez MC, Bussmann J, Janssen W, Horemans H, Chastin S, Heijenbrok M, Stam H. Accelerometric assessment of different dimensions of natural walking during the first year after stroke: recovery of amount, distribution, quality and speed of walking. J Rehabil Med. 2015;47(8):714–21.

Shumway-Cook A, Woollacott MH, Rachwani J, Santamaria V. Abnormal mobility In: Motor control: translating research into clinical practice (Chapter 12). 6th ed. Philadelphia: Lippincott Williams & Wilkins; 2023a. p. 407–39.

Shumway-Cook A, Woollacott MH, Rachwani J, Santamaria V. Development of mobility. In: Motor control: translating research into clinical practice (Chapter 13). 6th ed. Philadelphia: Lippincott Williams & Wilkins; 2023b. p. 367–88.

Snijders AH, van de Warrenburg BP, Giladi N, Bloem BR. Neurological gait disorders in elderly people: clinical approach and classification. Lancet Neurol. 2007;6(1):63–74.

Takakusaki K. Neurophysiology of gait: from the spinal cord to the frontal lobe. Mov Disord. 2013;28(11):1483–91.

Takakusaki K, Tomita N, Yano M. Substrates for normal gait and pathophysiology of gait disturbances with respect to the basal ganglia dysfunction. J Neurol. 2008;255(Suppl 4):19–29.

Toulotte C, Thevenon A, Fabre C. Effects of training and detraining on the static and dynamic balance in elderly fallers and non-fallers: a pilot study. Disabil Rehabil. 2006;28(2):125–33.

Trompetto C, Currà A, Puce L, Mori L, Serrati C, Fattapposta F, Abbruzzese G, Marinelli L. Spastic dystonia in stroke subjects: prevalence and features of the neglected phenomenon of the upper motor neuron syndrome. Clin Neurophysiol. 2019;130(4):521–7.

Wolf SL, Catlin PA, Ellis M, Archer AL, Morgan B, Piacentino A. Assessing Wolf motor function test as outcome measure for research in patients after stroke. Stroke. 2001;32(7):1635–9.

Yu WH, Liu WY, Wong AM, Wang TC, Li YC, Lien HY. Effect of forced use of the lower extremity on gait performance and mobility of post-acute stroke patients. J Phys Ther Sci. 2015;27(2):421–5.

3 Normal Gait

3.1 Definition of Gait

Gait is a process that involves moving from one place to another by repetitively and reciprocally stepping across the ground using the two lower limbs. The gait cycle begins at the initial contact of one foot and ends at the next initial contact of the same foot. It is helpful to use the gait cycle, its periods, and phases to comprehend gait as joint angles and muscle actions repeat at specific times during the gait cycle.

3.2 Requirements of Normal Gait

Normal gait should be safe, energy-efficient, and adaptable to individual needs. For safe gait, a good balance ability (postural stability) is essential. Energy-efficient gait requires the coordinated contraction of many muscles in the body (kinematics) and the optimal movement of body segments (kinetics). This optimal movement of body segments not only creates a favorable appearance but also minimizes the risk of injury.

3.3 Energy Conservation

To achieve optimal endurance, the energy cost of walking should be less than 50% of maximal aerobic capacity (Waters et al. 1999). In normal walking that occurs at a speed of 82 m/min, the energy cost of walking is 38% of the maximum aerobic capacity (Waters et al. 1999). Minimizing energy consumption during gait is crucial, especially for the elderly and individuals with cardiopulmonary problems. Abnormal gait patterns, such as slow gait speed, asymmetric gait, and abnormal joint motion, can increase the energy cost of gait. Therefore, preventing and correcting abnormal gait patterns is one of the most important goals of gait training. Several mechanisms are employed to reduce the energy cost of gait, including the conversion of energy, minimizing the movement of the center of mass, optimizing muscle contraction, and energy storage and release.

3.3.1 Conversion of Energy

Despite employing various mechanisms to reduce the movement of the center of mass, some degree of vertical and lateral movement of the center of mass is inevitable. To reduce energy costs, a crucial mechanism is the conversion of energy. This involves the transfer of energy between kinetic and gravitational potential energy and may be the most important mechanism for reducing the metabolic cost of walking (Fig. 3.1). The maximum recovery of mechanical energy through the transfer of energy between gravitational potential and kinetic energy during walking was found to be around two-thirds (Cavagna et al. 1976; Dewolf et al. 2017).

Efficient energy transfer requires moving the center of mass in a smooth, sinusoidal fashion.

Y.-S. Lee, *Task Oriented Gait Training*, https://doi.org/10.1007/978-981-97-3348-4_3

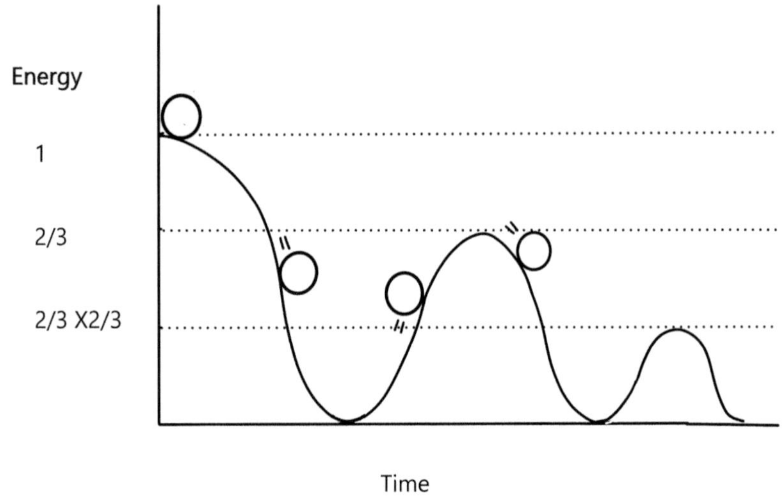

Fig. 3.1 Conversion of energy

The movement of the body during the stance phase of gait can be visualized as an inverted pendulum. The center of mass of the body rotates on the foot, progressing through different rocker phases.

Heel rocker phase: Initially, the rotation occurs on the heel of the foot. This phase involves the initial contact of the foot with the ground, and the body's center of mass rotates over the heel to create a rocking motion.

Ankle rocker phase: Following the heel rocker phase, the rotation transitions to the ankle joint. During this phase, the ankle joint allows the body's center of mass to continue its forward movement while maintaining stability.

Forefoot rocker phase: After the ankle rocker phase, the rotation shifts to the forefoot. This phase enables the body's center of mass to progress further, with the forefoot acting as a pivot point.

Toe rocker phase: Finally, the rotation occurs at the toes of the foot. The toe rocker phase helps propel the body forward and prepares for the swing phase of gait.

These sequential rotations that occur at different parts of the foot allow for an efficient transfer of energy and forward progression during the stance phase of gait, resembling the movement of an inverted pendulum.

3.3.2 Minimizing Movement of the Center of Mass

In normal walking, the center of mass of the human body moves both vertically, up and down, and laterally, side to side. Without modifying mechanisms, the center of mass moves approximately 9.5 cm vertically and 8 cm laterally (Saunders et al. 1953). Saunders, Inman, and Eberhart identified six determinants that reduce the vertical and lateral movement of the center of mass in gait (Saunders et al. 1953). However, recent studies conducted using modern technology have revealed that pelvic rotation has little effect on the vertical displacement of the body's mass (Kerrigan et al. 2001). Similarly, pelvic tilt and knee flexion were found to have virtually no effect on the vertical movement of the center of mass (Gard and Childress 1999). These three determinants likely contribute to shock absorption.

In contrast, the foot and ankle mechanisms are major contributing factors in reducing the vertical movement of the center of mass (Gard and Childress 2001). The neutral ankle position at initial contact and heel rise at terminal stance decrease the downward movement of the center of mass. Additionally, the foot-ankle rocker can facilitate forward progression (Gard and Childress 2001). To minimize lateral movement of the center of mass, it must be positioned outside the base of support during single-limb support. Taking a step forward is necessary to maintain balance during single-limb support. Considering these facts, dynamic balance training should be utilized to regain gait ability.

The amount of displacement of the center of mass is dependent on walking velocity (Orendurff et al. 2004). At slow gait speeds, there is an increased lateral movement of the center of mass, placing a greater burden on mediolateral stability. This may explain why people with slow gait speeds tend to fall laterally and sustain injuries to the femur. Conversely, at fast walking speeds, there is an increased vertical movement of the center of mass.

3.3.3 Optimization of Muscle Contraction

In normal gait, each muscle is activated at a specific time and intensity to match the demands of the gait. If there is co-contraction or unnecessary muscle contraction, this can increase the energy cost of gait and interfere with normal gait.

3.3.4 Energy Storage and Release

In the pre-swing phase of gait, there is plantar flexion with minimal electromyography (EMG) activity while tendon recoil provides the force for ankle plantar flexion. However, there is debate about the role of ankle plantar flexors.

3.4 Adaptation to Need

For gait to be considered normal, it should meet specific needs. This includes navigating diverse terrains such as inclines, stairs, curbs, uneven ground, moving surfaces, and slippery surfaces. If there are obstacles in the path, individuals must be able to negotiate them by stepping over or stepping around obstacles. Additionally, adaptation to external threats requires perceptual and cognitive functions to detect and plan for the avoidance of dangers such as slipping, tripping, or colliding.

3.5 Velocity of Gait

With an increase in gait velocity, both cadence (the number of steps taken in 1 min) and step length (the distance covered by one foot in one gait cycle) increase. As gait velocity increases, the duration of the gait cycle shortens, with a more significant decrease in double-limb stance time. Eventually, once a certain gait velocity is reached, double-limb stance time disappears completely as gait transitions into running. Conversely, at lower gait velocities, the duration of the gait cycle increases, with a more substantial increase in the double-limb stance period. The energy cost of gait follows a U-shaped curve, with the most efficient gait velocity aligning with the gait speed that individuals find most comfortable. Given the importance of energy conversion, sufficient gait velocity is necessary to leverage the advantages of momentum for the sake of energy conversion. Achieving a steady velocity in gait typically requires one to three steps, depending on the magnitude of the velocity.

3.6 Toe Out

The axis of the foot is different from the direction of progression, which can potentially lead to severe ankle joint damage. When walking, this issue is resolved through the motion of the subtalar joint. Eversion of the subtalar joint leads to internal rotation of the tibia, aligning the rotation of the ankle axis with the direction of progression. In elderly individuals, toe out is often increased, possibly serving as a compensation mechanism to enhance stability during times of one-legged support.

3.7 Stride Width

Stride width refers to the distance between the centers of the two heels, measured perpendicular to the direction of progression during gait. The stride width for men is approximately 8 cm, while for women, it is around 7 cm (Murray et al. 1964). Increasing stride width necessitates a greater lateral displacement of the center of mass, resulting in an increased energy cost of gait.

3.8 Gait Cycle

3.8.1 Division of the Gait Cycle

The gait cycle consists of two main phases: the stance period and the swing period. During the stance period, one specific foot is on the ground, and at a self-selected gait speed, it constitutes approximately 60% of the gait cycle. In the swing period, the same foot is in the air, and in normal gait, it makes up about 40% of the gait cycle. However, the duration of these periods varies with gait speed.

In the stance period, the most important tasks are supporting the body's weight, maintaining balance, and moving the center of mass forward. In the swing period, the primary task is advancing the swing leg and repositioning the limb for weight acceptance.

Within the gait cycle, there are two instances in which both feet are on the ground, a period known as double-limb stance. These are the initial double-limb stance and the terminal double-limb stance (Fig. 3.2). The initial double-limb stance includes the initial contact and loading response phases. On the other hand, mid-stance and terminal stance represent stance periods with single-limb support. The terminal double-limb stance is the same as the pre-swing phase. The swing period consists of the initial swing phase, the mid-swing phase, and the terminal swing phase.

Understanding the gait cycle, including the motion of body segments and the activation of muscles throughout its varying phases, is crucial for effective gait training.

3.8.2 Initial Contact Phase

Initial contact covers 0–2% of the gait cycle and is part of the initial double-limb stance period.

The critical events during initial contact are the initial contact itself, the initiation of the heel rocker, and shock absorption.

Initial contact begins with the foot making contact with the ground, usually starting with the heel. However, some people may make initial contact with other parts of the foot, which can lead to the loss of the heel rocker and an increase in the energy cost of gait.

During initial contact, the hip is flexed to 20° to achieve adequate step length, and the knee is fully extended to accommodate proper step length. Incomplete knee extension can result in decreased step length, reduced gait velocity, and increased energy cost.

The ankle remains in a neutral position to facilitate the heel rocker and the forward pulling

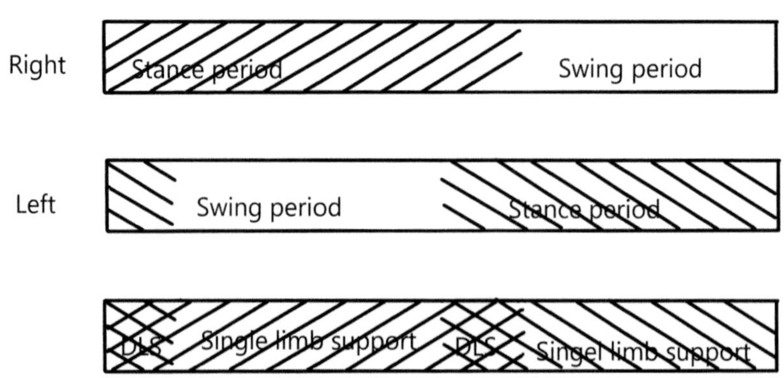

Fig. 3.2 Division of the gait cycle. *DLS* double-limb stance

of the tibia. The heel rocker is essential for the smooth anterior movement of the tibia. As the ground reaction force vector passes posterior to the ankle joint, the foot is plantar—flexed from neutral to 2.5° by the end of the initial contact. At the moment of initial contact, the subtalar joint is in a neutral position.

Ankle plantar flexion and subtalar eversion contribute to shock absorption. However, improper foot alignment, which leads to the absence of the heel rocker, can negatively impact the forward progression of the body, resulting in decreased gait velocity and increased energy cost.

During this phase, the activation of hip extensors, knee extensors, and ankle dorsiflexors is required. Hip extensor muscles are necessary to restrain the forward movement of the head, arms, and trunk segments. Eccentric contraction of the tibialis anterior decelerates ankle plantar flexion and draws the tibia forward. The motion of the ankle joint is controlled by the eccentric contraction of the ankle dorsiflexor, which draws the tibia forward and contributes to shock absorption.

3.8.3 Loading Response Phase

The loading response phase covers 2–12% of the gait cycle and is part of the initial double-stance period. It terminates when the other foot is lifted for the swing phase. During this phase, controlled knee flexion is an important factor for shock absorption.

The critical events of the loading response phase include the heel rocker, controlled ankle plantar flexion, and controlled knee flexion.

For individuals who make initial contact with their heel, the stance limb rotates continuously around the heel, facilitating the progression of the entire body in this phase (heel rocker). The ankle joint undergoes plantar flexion from 2.5 to a peak of 5° by the midpoint of the loading phase via eccentric contraction of the pretibial muscles. By the end of the loading phase, the ankle is dorsiflexed to a neutral position.

Eccentric contraction of the pretibial muscles delays the plantar flexion of the ankle joint and draws the tibia forward. If there is no ankle plantar flexion, the tibia moves too far anteriorly, thus increasing the demand on the quadriceps. Eccentric contraction of the quadriceps decelerates the rate of knee flexion, which is essential for absorbing the impact of foot strike and advancing the femur forward. By the end of this phase, the knee joint is flexed to 20°, which is a key mechanism for shock absorption. Severe weakness in the knee extensors can result in the knee joint buckling, leading to falls. To prevent this, individuals with weakness of their knee extensors should use genu recurvatum to establish knee joint stability. The loss of knee flexion leads to increased impact on the body and may increase the energy cost of gait.

During this period, the subtalar joint becomes everted to 5°, which rotates the tibia internally and aligns the axis of the ankle joint with the direction of progression. The use of ankle-foot orthosis increases the burden on the quadriceps and inhibits subtalar eversion. Some people with ankle-foot orthosis may find walking more difficult due to compromised stance stability and increased demand on the quadriceps.

To control trunk flexion, single-joint hip extensors (the gluteus maximus and adductor magnus) and low-level hamstrings reach their peak activity. As the weight shifts to the leg during the loading period, the pelvis of the trailing limb drops. To control pelvic drop and aid in shock absorption, intense eccentric contraction of abductor muscles (the gluteus medius, upper gluteus maximus, and posterior tensor fascia lata) is required.

3.8.4 Mid-Stance Phase

The mid-stance phase covers 12–31% of the gait cycle and is part of the single-limb support period. Critical events during the mid-stance phase include controlled ankle dorsiflexion, knee extension, and coronal plane hip stabilization.

In the mid-stance phase, the body rotates around the ankle joint, known as the ankle rocker, and dorsiflexes from neutral to 5° dorsiflexion by the end of the mid-stance phase. This dorsiflexion contributes to shock absorption.

Eccentric contraction of ankle plantar flexors, mainly due to the action of the soleus muscle, controls the speed of forward movement of the tibia and provides stability for knee extension. Reduced flexibility of the ankle joint can interfere with the ankle rocker, leading to decreased gait speed and increased energy cost.

During the mid-stance phase, eversion of the subtalar joint is controlled via activity of the tibialis posterior and soleus, keeping it at 5°. Although knee extensor activation is required during the early mid-stance, knee extensor activity ceases by the middle of the mid-stance phase.

To control pelvic drop, eccentric contraction occurs in the hip abductor muscles of the stance limb. If the hip abductor action is inadequate, compensatory mechanisms, such as leaning the trunk toward the supporting leg, may become necessary.

3.8.5 Terminal Stance Phase

The terminal stance phase covers 31–50% of the gait cycle and is part of the single-limb support period. It begins with the heel lift of the stance foot and ends at the contact of the other foot with the ground. During this phase, the body rotates on the forefoot, known as the forefoot rocker.

Critical events of the terminal stance phase include controlled dorsiflexion with heel rise and trailing limb posture.

The ankle joint experiences 5°–10° of dorsiflexion due to stretching of the Achilles tendon at 45% of the gait cycle. The ankle joint then remains in this position throughout the final 5% of the terminal stance. Ankle dorsiflexion facilitates the progression of the body's center of mass. During this phase, the heel is raised to 3.5 cm by the end of the terminal stance phase, which is the main source of tibial advancement.

Strong activity of the soleus and gastrocnemius muscles locks the ankle during the terminal stance, causing the foot to rotate on the forefoot rocker. During the late terminal stance phase, eversion of the subtalar joint is progressively reduced, reaching 2° by the end of the terminal stance. Decreased eversion, mediated by the peroneal muscles and tibialis posterior, reduces the mobility of the midtarsal joint and provides foot stability.

3.8.6 Pre-Swing Phase

The pre-swing phase covers 50–62% of the gait cycle and is part of the second double-stance period.

Critical events during the pre-swing phase include the toe rocker and knee flexion reaching 40°.

This phase is a preparation for the swing phase in which ankle plantar flexion leads to the flexion of the knee joint and a reduction in hip extension. As weight transfers to the other leg, the ankle joint plantar flexes from 10° dorsiflexion to a peak of 15° plantar flexion. Elastic recoil and active contraction of the plantar flexors thrust the tibia forward, leading to knee flexion reaching up to 40°, which in turn prepares the limb for the swing phase.

The lack of ankle plantar flexion requires increased hip flexion of the trailing leg, which can be more challenging for individuals with weak hip flexors.

Much of the energy needed to initiate the swing phase is generated during the pre-swing phase.

Toward the end of the pre-swing phase, activation of the tibialis anterior is initiated, decelerating ankle plantar flexion and preparing for ankle dorsiflexion during the initial swing for foot lift. During this pre-swing phase, the leg rotates around the toes, an action known as the toe rocker. Limited range of motion at the metatarsophalangeal joint can interfere with the toe rocker, reducing step length and increasing energy consumption.

Additionally, during the pre-swing phase, the subtalar joint progressively inverts and achieves a neutral position.

3.8.7 Initial Swing Phase

The initial swing phase covers 62–75% of the gait cycle and is the initial part of the swing period. It begins with lifting the foot from the ground and terminates when the swing foot is opposite to the stance foot. Critical events during the initial swing phase include knee flexion and hip flexion.

At a normal walking speed, limb advancement may be passive, relying on the ankle's propulsive mechanics. However, at slower walking speeds, limb advancement requires the activation of hip flexors. Since most people with gait problems walk slowly, the activity of hip flexors is necessary for progression. Hip flexion is primarily provided by the iliacus muscle and is augmented by the gracilis and sartorius. Weak hip flexors may lead to compensatory movements such as external hip rotation (compensation by hip adductors) or circumduction.

During the initial swing, the activation of hip and knee flexors, as well as ankle dorsiflexors, is needed for the sake of foot clearance. The knee joint flexes from 40° to 60°, with knee flexion being more critical than ankle dorsiflexion for achieving toe clearance. The ankle joint dorsiflexes from 15° of plantar flexion to 5° of plantar flexion by the end of the initial swing phase.

3.8.8 Mid-Swing Phase

The mid-swing phase covers 75–87% of the gait cycle and represents the middle of the swing period. It begins when the swing foot is opposite of the stance foot and terminates when the tibia of the swing limb is in a vertical position. Critical events during the mid-swing phase include ankle dorsiflexion and hip flexion.

For adequate foot clearance, dorsiflexion of the ankle joint is required during mid-swing. The ankle joint dorsiflexes from 5° of plantar flexion to a neutral position at 79% of the gait cycle. After this, the ankle maintains this position. The activity of the ankle pretibial muscles decreases during the latter half of the mid-swing phase. When there is inadequate ankle dorsiflexion, compensatory movements, such as exaggerated hip flexion, may be necessary.

3.8.9 Terminal Swing Phase

The terminal swing phase covers 87–100% of the gait cycle and represents the terminal part of the swing period. It begins when the tibia is in a vertical position and terminates when the foot contacts the ground. Critical events during the terminal swing phase include hip deceleration, knee extension, and ankle dorsiflexion.

During terminal swing, it is necessary to have the activation of hip extensors, knee extensors, and ankle dorsiflexors. Hamstring activity is also needed to slow down the forward rotation of the thigh in preparation for foot contact with the ground. Adequate knee extension is required for limb advancement while maintaining ankle dorsiflexion at a neutral position is crucial to prepare for heel contact and the heel rocker.

3.9 Summary

Normal gait is characterized by several key principles: safety, energy efficiency, and adaptability to different needs. Achieving these principles requires a combination of factors related to balance, kinematics, and kinetics.

Safe gait relies on good balance and postural stability. This involves maintaining equilibrium throughout the gait cycle to prevent falls and injuries.

Several mechanisms are employed to reduce the energy cost of gait, including the conversion of energy, the minimizing of movement of center of mass, the optimization of muscle contraction, and energy storage and release.

Normal gait should be able to adapt to various conditions and terrains, including inclines, stairs, uneven ground, and slippery surfaces. Perceptual and cognitive functions are required to detect and respond to external threats.

During the gait cycle, joint angles and muscle actions repeat at specific times. Understanding the gait cycle, including the motion of body segments and the activation of muscles throughout its phases, is crucial for effective gait training.

References

Cavagna GA, Thys H, Zamboni A. The sources of external work in level walking and running. J Physiol. 1976;262(3):639–57.

Dewolf AH, Ivanenko YP, Lacquaniti F, Willems PA. Pendular energy transduction within the step during human walking on slopes at different speeds. PLoS One. 2017;12(10):e0186963.

Gard SA, Childress DS. The influence of stance-phase knee flexion on the vertical displacement of the trunk during normal walking. Arch Phys Med Rehabil. 1999;80(1):26–32.

Gard SA, Childress DS. What determines the vertical displacement of the body during normal walking? JPO J Prosthet Orthotics. 2001;13(3):64–7.

Kerrigan DC, Riley PO, Lelas JL, Croce UD. Quantification of pelvic rotation as a determinant of gait. Arch Phys Med Rehabil. 2001;82(2):217–20.

Murray MP, Drought AB, Kory RC. Walking patterns of normal men. J Bone Jt Surg. 1964;46A:335–60.

Orendurff MS, Segal AD, Klute GK, Berge JS, Rohr ES, Kadel NJ. The effect of walking speed on center of mass displacement. J Rehabil Res Dev. 2004;41(6A):829–34.

Saunders JB, Inman VT, Eberhart HD. The major determinants in normal and pathological gait. J Bone Jt Surg Am. 1953;35-A(3):543–58.

Waters RL, Mulroy S, S. The energy expenditure of normal and pathologic gait. Gait Posture. 1999;9(3):207–31.

4 Abnormal Gait

4.1 Effects of Abnormal Gait

Abnormal gait increases the movement of the center of mass, leading to inefficient energy conversion and a slower walking speed. As a result, it increases energy consumption and the risk of injury. In the short term, it can lead to falls, and in the long term, abnormal gait can result in musculoskeletal problems (i.e., cumulative stress injuries).

4.2 Evaluation of Abnormal Gait

One impairment can result in many abnormal gait patterns, and in many cases, a single person can have multiple impairments and disabilities causing abnormal gait. While it is easy to identify abnormal gait, pinpointing the main cause can be rather challenging. Even if two cases of abnormal gait look similar, the underlying causes may differ. Proper assessment is necessary to identify the cause of abnormal gait and manage it effectively.

4.3 Causes of Abnormal Gait

4.3.1 Weakness

4.3.1.1 Hip Flexor Weakness

Hip flexor weakness impacts the ability to advance the swing limb, resulting in poor toe clearance and shortened step length. People with hip flexor weakness compensate using several methods. Firstly, they use posterior pelvic tilt and the abdominal muscles to advance the swing limb. Secondly, they might use circumduction, which involves hip hiking, forward pelvic rotation, and hip abduction to advance the swing limb. Thirdly, some individuals might use contralateral limb vaulting. Finally, leaning the trunk to the contralateral side is another common compensation method. These compensative methods result in a poor appearance and increased energy consumption.

4.3.1.2 Hip Extensor Weakness

Hip extensors are crucial for controlling the forward movement of the head, arms, and trunk during gait. At initial contact, hip extensors should control hip flexion momentum, which increases with gait speed. To compensate for hip extensor weakness, people lean tend to their trunks backward, thus moving the center of mass to the posterior and reducing the need for hip extensor activation. However, this compensation might increase the risk of falling. Therefore, individuals with hip extensor weakness, especially those with poor balance, must reduce their gait speed, leading to increased energy consumption.

4.3.1.3 Hip Abductor Weakness

Abnormal gait caused by hip abductor weakness is velocity-dependent, but the relationship is actually inverse to one's walking speed. Remarkable abnormalities are more evident at slow walking speeds, while they become less pronounced at faster walk-

Y.-S. Lee, *Task Oriented Gait Training*, https://doi.org/10.1007/978-981-97-3348-4_4

ing velocities. The weakness of hip abductor muscles—the gluteus medius, minimus, and tensor fasciae latae—contributes to pelvic drop on the swing side. Mild hip abductor muscle weakness leads to contralateral pelvic drop during the stance period (noncompensated gluteus medius gait). Severe weakness causes ipsilateral trunk tilting (thus compensating the gluteus medius gait). When walking at a slow pace, the demand for hip abductor muscle contraction and mediolateral movement of the center of mass increases. Since people with gait disabilities tend to walk slowly, this exacerbates the problem and leads to increased energy consumption. In addition, hip abductor muscle weakness results in instability in the frontal plane, increasing the risk of falls and thus hip fractures in the elderly population (Krebs et al. 1998).

4.3.1.4 Hip Internal Rotator Weakness

Weakness of the hip internal rotators creates increased difficulty in controlling the external rotation of the femur and leads to external rotation of the lower limb. This leads to a poor appearance when walking and an increased energy cost.

4.3.1.5 Knee Extensor Weakness and Paresis

Weak knee extensors make it difficult to control knee flexion during the loading and mid-stance phase. Individuals with weak knee extensors compensate by hyperextending their knee (genu recurvatum) during the mid-stance phase. Knee hyperextension shifts the center of mass anterior to the knee joint axis, and stability at the knee relies on passive joint components (like the joint capsule and ligaments). Knee hyperextension interferes with hip flexion in the pre-swing and initial swing phase. Another compensation for knee extensor weakness is forward trunk lean, which shifts the body vector anterior to the knee joint and further exacerbates knee hyperextension. In cases of paresis, controlled eccentric contraction is more difficult to obtain than concentric contraction. Since controlled knee flexion is necessary during the loading response, individuals with poor knee extensor control also compensate by utilizing knee hyperextension.

4.3.1.6 Ankle Dorsiflexor Weakness

The degree of ankle dorsiflexor weakness leads to different abnormalities. Moderate weakness causes foot slap or whole-foot contact at the initial contact phase. Severe weakness results in forefoot contact at the initial contact and poor foot clearance during the mid-swing. Poor foot clearance due to ankle dorsiflexor weakness disrupts swing limb advancement, leading to compensatory behaviors such as steppage gait (exaggerated hip flexion), the trunk leaning to the contralateral side, and hip circumduction. The loss of initial heel contact (whole foot or forefoot) diminishes the heel rocker and decreases progression of the center of mass, consequently leading to an increase in energy consumption.

4.3.1.7 Ankle Evertor Weakness

Ankle evertor weakness exacerbates ankle inversion for the swing limb. Landing in an excessively inverted position makes weight-bearing more difficult and increases the risk of ankle inversion injuries.

4.3.1.8 Ankle Plantar Flexor Weakness/Paresis

Weak ankle plantar flexors make ankle plantar flexion during pre-swing impossible, thus interfering with hip flexion during pre-swing. Individuals with ankle plantar flexor paresis have difficulty controlling tibia forward advancement in the mid-stance phase, which often causes them to compensate through the use of knee hyperextension. Plantar paresis is a significant cause of knee hyperextension in individuals with stroke. Since ankle plantar flexion is a primary source of walking energy, its impairment leads to a slower walking speed and reduced endurance.

4.3.2 Loss of Flexibility

4.3.2.1 Causes of Loss of Flexibility

Loss of flexibility can be caused by a variety of factors, including soft tissue contracture, spasticity (or spastic dystonia), and bony deformity. Clinically, it is challenging to distinguish between contracture and severe spasticity.

4.3.2.2 Effects of Loss of Flexibility

Loss of flexibility limits the forward movement of the body during the stance period, thus reducing foot clearance, progression, and proper foot placement during the swing period (Shumway-Cook et al. 2023).

4.3.2.3 Hip Flexion Contracture

Contracture of the hip flexor interferes with the advancement of the center of mass. It leads to insufficient hip extension in the terminal stance phase, resulting in a shortened step length and slower gait speed. In severe contractures, achieving vertical trunk alignment becomes impossible, leading to an anteriorly tilted trunk, with knee flexion acting as a common compensation. The anteriorly tilted trunk increases the demand on the hip extensors and significantly increases energy consumption. Knee flexion further increases the demand on the quadriceps muscles during mid-stance and subsequently increases energy consumption.

4.3.2.4 Hip Adductor Spasticity

Hip adductor spasticity is a common issue in children with diplegic cerebral palsy and can manifest as a scissoring gait. It reduces the base of support, resulting in poor stability, and in severe cases, it can even impede the forward movement of the swing limb.

4.3.2.5 Quadriceps Spasticity

During the stance period, quadriceps spasticity can lead to knee hyperextension. In the swing period, it can result in a stiff knee gait. This is commonly observed in hemiparetic stroke patients and children with cerebral palsy, where decreased knee flexion during swing may necessitate hip circumduction as a form of compensation.

4.3.2.6 Knee Flexion Contracture/Hamstring Spasticity

Knee flexion contracture/hamstring spasticity is a frequent problem in children with diplegic cerebral palsy and presents as a crouched gait pattern. This condition interferes with full knee extension in the terminal stance phase and decreases step length. Excessive knee flexion during the stance phase increases the demand on the quadriceps muscles to prevent limb collapse, significantly increasing energy costs. The effects are particularly prominent when flexion exceeds 15° (Perry and Burnfield 2010, pp. 165–174).

4.3.2.7 Ankle Plantar Flexor Contracture/Spasticity

Ankle plantar flexor contracture/spasticity is a common problem in children with spastic cerebral palsy. In individuals with this condition, initial contact with the heel is impossible, leading to a loss of the heel rocker. This, in turn, impacts forward progression and results in increased energy consumption. In the mid-stance, contracture of the ankle plantar flexor impedes the forward rotation of the lower leg, potentially causing knee hyperextension. Severe contracture or spasticity can cause mid-stance knee hyperextension that continues into the pre-swing phase. During the swing period, ankle plantar flexor contracture/spasticity reduces foot clearance (toe drag), impedes progression, and affects proper foot placement. Additionally, severe spasticity in the triceps surae and posterior tibialis muscles can lead to foot inversion and an increased risk of ankle inversion injury.

4.3.3 Pain

Individuals experiencing pain in the lower back or a lower limb exhibit a variety of compensatory methods, including decreased gait velocity, reduced weight-bearing time on the afflicted limb, avoidance of forced foot contact, reduced joint excursion, and diminished joint compression forces.

4.3.4 Sensory Disorders

4.3.4.1 Impaired Somatosensory

Individuals with impaired somatosensory function walk slowly and have an increased risk of falls. Moderate sensory loss leads to forceful initial contact and knee wobbling. In cases of profound somatosensory loss, individuals may need to visually monitor their lower extremities to maintain balance during gait.

4.3.4.2 Impaired Vision

People with visual deficits also walk more slowly. Even at a reduced walking speed, detecting obstacles and potential threats in order to adjust gait and avoid injury become difficult.

4.3.4.3 Impaired Vestibular Sensory

Aminoglycoside use can damage the vestibular sensory organ. Individuals with vestibular deficits walk slowly and experience prolonged gait cycle times mainly due to increased double support time. Due to difficulties in regard to head stabilization, those with impaired vestibular sensory input minimize head motion, leading to challenges in gaze stabilization and contributing to impaired vision.

4.3.5 Balance Problems

4.3.5.1 Cerebellar Ataxia

Cerebellar ataxia occurs when the cerebellum or related structures are damaged. Individuals with cerebellar ataxia exhibit a wide-based gait, resembling a person walking on a rocking boat, often causing them to appear intoxicated. While many people with ataxia have increased step width, some studies have reported no increase in step width in people with chronic ataxia (Seidel and Krebs 2002).

4.3.5.2 Cautious Gait

In elderly individuals with gait disabilities, balance problems are often the most frequent and significant cause of gait disability. Those with poor balance exhibit slow walking speeds, reduced step and stride lengths, longer stride durations, increased gait cycle variability, reduced joint motion, and increased step width. Many individuals with balance issues display excessive flexion of the trunk, knee, and elbow (Snijders et al. 2007).

4.4 Classification of Abnormal Gait by Gait Pattern (Kinematics)

4.4.1 Causes of Abnormal Gait Patterns

While it is easy to identify abnormal gait patterns, identifying the primary cause of an abnormal gait is more challenging. Even though two cases of abnormal gait may appear similar, their underlying causes can differ significantly. Proper assessment is necessary to identify the cause of abnormal gait and manage it effectively.

4.4.2 Abnormal Movement of the Trunk

4.4.2.1 Importance of Vertical Trunk

A vertically aligned trunk is vital for the sake of energy conservation, flexibility, and aesthetics. Gravity's effects on the trunk are minimized in the vertical position, which should be maintained throughout all phases of the gait cycle.

4.4.2.2 Side Lean

Trunk leaning toward the stance limb can be caused by hip abductor weakness, hip flexor weakness, or pain in the hip joint. Forceful contraction aimed at supporting the pelvis increases hip joint compression and hip pain, leading individuals to lean their trunks toward the stance limb. Trunk lean toward the stance limb can improve foot clearance in individuals with hip flexor weakness.

4.4.2.3 Forward Lean

Forward trunk lean occurs in cases of hip flexion contracture, ankle plantar flexor contracture (or spasticity), weak hip extensors, and when walking with a walker.

4.4.2.4 Backward Lean

People with weak hip extensors struggle to control the forward movement of the head, arms, and trunk (HAT) at heel strike. This can be compensated by slowing gait velocity and placing the center of mass posterior to the hip joints during the stance phase. A backward trunk lean can also occur as a compensatory method for hip flexor weakness during the swing period.

4.4.3 Abnormal Movement of the Pelvis

4.4.3.1 Anterior Pelvic Tilt

Anterior pelvic tilt can be caused by hip flexion contracture (or spasticity), hip extensor weakness, and abdominal muscle weakness.

4.4.3.2 Posterior Pelvic Tilt

Posterior pelvic tilt can be caused by hamstring muscle contracture, lower back pain, and hip flexor weakness.

4.4.3.3 Contralateral Pelvic Drop

Contralateral pelvic drop can be caused by hip adductor contracture, hip adductor spasticity, and hip abductor weakness.

4.4.3.4 Ipsilateral Pelvic Drop

Ipsilateral pelvic drop can be caused by weakness in the calf muscles and when one leg is shorter than the contralateral side.

4.4.3.5 Pelvic Hike

Pelvic hike can be caused by limited hip flexion at the mid-swing phase, limited knee flexion at the initial swing phase, and limited ankle dorsiflexion at the mid-swing phase when it occurs to facilitate foot clearance.

4.4.4 Abnormal Movement of the Hip

4.4.4.1 Hip Circumduction

Hip circumduction involves hip hiking, forward pelvic rotation, and hip abduction. Individuals with weak hip flexors can use hip circumduction to advance the swing limb.

4.4.4.2 Excessive Hip Abduction

Excessive hip abduction can be caused by hip abductor contracture, inadequate hip flexion, leg length discrepancy (i.e., when one leg is longer than the other), medial brim knee-ankle-foot orthosis, a transfemoral prosthesis causing pain, or hip joint problems.

4.4.4.3 Excessive Hip Adduction

Excessive hip adduction can result from hip adductor contracture, hip adductor spasticity, hip flexor weakness, or hip abductor weakness.

4.4.4.4 Excessive Hip Flexion

Excessive hip flexion can be due to hip flexion contracture, hip flexor spasticity, contracture of the iliotibial band, hip pain, excessive ankle plantar flexion at the mid-swing phase (when acting as compensation), excessive knee flexion, and ankle dorsiflexion during the stance period (when acting as compensation).

4.4.4.5 Limited Hip Flexion

Limited hip flexion can be caused by hip pain, hamstring spasticity, hip extensor weakness (when acting as compensation), and hip flexor weakness.

4.4.4.6 Past Retract

Past retract refers to excessive hip flexion and extension after hip flexion. This can be caused by weakness of the quadriceps, leading to passive knee extension using hip movement.

4.4.4.7 Excessive Hip External Rotation

Excessive hip external rotation can result from hip arthritis, hip external rotation contracture, overactivity of the gluteus maximus, weakness of hip internal rotators, ankle plantar flexion contracture (when acting as compensation), and when one limb is longer than the other.

4.4.4.8 Excessive Hip Internal Rotation

Excessive hip internal rotation can be caused by femoral anteversion, contracture of the hip internal rotator, spasticity of the hip internal rotator, or weakness of the quadriceps (when acting as compensation).

4.4.5 Abnormal Movement of the Knee

4.4.5.1 Genu Recurvatum (Knee Hyperextension)

Knee hyperextension in the stance period can result from spasticity of the quadriceps or ankle plantar flexor, or from contracture of the ankle joint or ankle plantar flexor muscles. Knee hyperextension can compensate for weakness of the knee extensors and ankle plantar flexors or poor control of knee extensors. Knee hyperextension in the pre-swing phase interferes with knee flexion for limb advancement, leading to slow swing limb progression and poor toe clearance. Persistent knee hyperextension can also cause knee joint injuries.

4.4.5.2 Limited Knee Flexion

Limited knee flexion can be due to contracture of the knee extensors, impaired proprioception, knee pain, primitive extension synergy, quadriceps spasticity, ankle plantar flexor spasticity, hip flexor weakness, or quadriceps weakness. Overactivity of the hamstrings can also restrict femur forward movement, resulting in limited knee flexion.

4.4.5.3 Excessive Knee Flexion

Excessive knee flexion can be caused by contracture of the knee flexors, knee pain, primitive flexion synergy, hamstrings spasticity, ankle plantar flexor weakness, or when one limb is longer than the other (anatomically or functionally).

4.4.5.4 Wobble

Wobble refers to alternating flexion and extension of the knee joint during the stance period. This can be caused by proprioceptive deficits, spastic clonus of the quadriceps, or ankle plantar flexor spasticity.

4.4.5.5 Excessive Valgus of the Knee Joint

Excessive valgus of the knee joint can be the result of knee joint deformities, ipsilateral abductor weakness, ipsilateral trunk lean, joint instability, or joint pain.

4.4.5.6 Excessive Varus of the Knee Joint

Excessive varus of the knee joint can be due to knee joint deformities, degenerative joint changes in the knee, joint instability, or joint pain.

4.4.6 Abnormal Movement of the Ankle

4.4.6.1 Excessive Plantar Flexion

Excessive plantar flexion can result from contracture of the ankle plantar flexors, spasticity of the ankle plantar flexors, weakness of the ankle dorsiflexors, or proprioceptive deficits. Excessive plantar flexion can reduce demand on the knee extensor muscles and may be used to compensate for weakness of the quadriceps.

4.4.6.2 Premature Heel Off

Premature heel off can occur due to excessive knee flexion, heel pain, or spasticity of the ankle plantar flexors. It can also serve as compensation for a shorter limb by assisting in contralateral foot clearance (vaulting).

4.4.6.3 Delayed Heel Off

Delayed heel off can be caused by forefoot pain, insufficient toe extension range of motion, or weakness of the ankle plantar flexors.

4.4.6.4 Lack of Heel Off

A lack of heel off can result from forefoot pain, inadequate toe extension range of motion, or weakness of the ankle plantar flexors.

4.4.6.5 Excess Ankle Dorsiflexion

Excess ankle dorsiflexion can occur due to weakness of the ankle plantar flexor muscles, an ankle locked in a neutral position, or accommodation for excessive hip flexion and knee flexion.

4.4.6.6 Prolonged Heel Only

Prolonged heel only can be caused by pain in the forefoot.

4.4.7 Abnormal Movement of the Subtalar Joint

4.4.7.1 Excess Eversion

Excess eversion can result from hypertonicity of the peroneal muscles, a valgus deformity, or weakness of the invertor muscles. Eversion can increase ankle dorsiflexion range of motion and may be used as compensation for ankle plantar flexor contracture.

4.4.7.2 Excess Inversion

Excess inversion can occur due to contracture of the invertor muscles, an equinovarus deformity, overactivity of the invertor muscles, or skeletal deformities.

4.4.8 Abnormal Movement of the Toes

4.4.8.1 Clawed Toe

Clawed toe can result from hypertonicity of the toe flexors or an imbalance in strength between intrinsic toe flexors and long toe flexors. Clawed toe can also be used as compensation for calf muscle weakness.

4.4.8.2 Excess Toe Extension

Excess toe extension can be due to hypertonicity of the toe extensors. Excessive toe extension may be used as compensation for weakness of the ankle dorsiflexors (tibialis anterior).

4.4.8.3 Limited Toe Extension

Limited toe extension can result from contracture of the toe flexors or forefoot pain.

4.5 Summary

Abnormal gait increases the movement of the center of mass, leading to inefficient energy conversion and a slow walking speed. As a result, it increases energy consumption and the risk of injury. In the short term, it can lead to falls, and in the long term, it can result in musculoskeletal problems.

Abnormal gait can be classified by its cause and kinematics. The same abnormal gait can arise from a variety of different impairments, and the same impairment can lead to different abnormal gaits depending on individual compensation mechanisms.

Primary impairments, such as weakness and paresis, can cause secondary impairments, such as contractures, and these secondary impairments can then lead to an abnormal gait.

For effective gait training, it is necessary to assess not only the gait pattern but also the impairments causing the abnormal gait.

References

Krebs DE, Jette AM, Assmann SF. Moderate exercise improves gait stability in disabled elders. Arch Phys Med Rehabil. 1998;79(12):1489–95.

Perry J, Burnfield J. Pathological mechanisms (Ch. 10). In: Gait analysis: normal and pathological function. 2nd ed. Thorofare: Slack Incorporated; 2010. p. 165–74.

Seidel B, Krebs DE. Base of support is not wider in chronic ataxic and unsteady patients. J Rehabil Med. 2002;34(6):288–92.

Shumway-Cook A, Woollacott MH, Rachwani J, Santamaria V. Abnormal mobility. In: Motor control: translating research into clinical practice (Chapter 15). 6th ed. Philadelphia: Lippincott Williams & Wilkins; 2023. p. 407–39.

Snijders AH, van de Warrenburg BP, Giladi N, Bloem BR. Neurological gait disorders in elderly people: clinical approach and classification. Lancet Neurol. 2007;6(1):63–74.

Part II

Evaluation

5 Assessment of Gait

5.1 Assessment of Participation

5.1.1 Self-Reported Measures

Social participation can be assessed using self-reported instruments such as the Craig Handicap Assessment and Reporting Techniques (mobility subscale) (Andrews 2012), the Mobility and Self-Care Questionnaire (Farin et al. 2007), and the Participation Survey/Mobility (Gray et al. 2006).

5.1.2 Ambulatory Monitoring

Ambulatory monitoring can serve as a useful outcome measure for gait training, offering insights into participation while simultaneously encouraging locomotor activity. Pedometers, simple devices used for counting steps, can also be utilized, though they have limitations as they are sensitive to gait speed and pattern (Cyarto et al. 2004). For conditions like Parkinson's disease that presents with abnormal gait patterns, waist-mounted devices tend to be more accurate than wrist-mounted ones (Wendel et al. 2018).

Nowadays, smartphone apps and activity logs also enable ambulatory monitoring.

5.2 Qualitative Tests Using Single Items

Gait assessment can utilize single-item tests such as walking straight, turning, and tandem gait. These tests evaluate whether the task is possible, the time needed to complete the task, the amount of sway, and foot alignment.

5.3 Classification of Gait Function

Several tests utilize gait classification, such as the Functional Ambulation Category and the Functional Ambulation Classification Scale. The Functional Ambulation Category assesses the level of assistance needed for walking (Wade 1992). The Functional Ambulation Classification Scale considers not only distance and the performance of various tasks (e.g., walking on tiptoes, walking on heels, tandem walking) but also gait appearance, such as whether a limp is present (Viosca et al. 2005). However, these tests have limitations due to their subjective nature and poor sensitivity.

Y.-S. Lee, *Task Oriented Gait Training*, https://doi.org/10.1007/978-981-97-3348-4_5

5.4 Quantitative Assessment Using Single Items

Spatiotemporal parameters are commonly used to evaluate gait function. Some parameters require high-tech equipment or cumbersome testing, such as analyzing step length, stride length, cadence, step width, single-limb support time, double-limb support time, and time of stance and swing phases. Hence, gait speed and distance covered in a specific time are the most frequently used measures.

5.4.1 Gait Velocity

Gait velocity is one of the most commonly used tests for evaluating gait function. It is considered the single best measure due to its simplicity, reliability, and lack of time consumption. Gait velocity is a composite measure that combines temporal (step frequency) and distance variables (step length) (Brandstater et al. 1983; Murray et al. 1970; Richards 1995). It also predicts community ambulation independence (Perry et al. 1995; Lord et al. 2004). Various other parameters are related to the this test, such as the type of pace, distance, and number of tests one takes.

Instructions for pace vary, encompassing such classifications as normal, slow, comfortable, self-selected, preferred (Menezes-Oliveira et al. 2021), and fastest speeds. Most individuals tend to walk at their preferred pace, which optimizes energy efficiency (Shumway-Cook et al. 2023b). Comfortable or preferred walking speeds minimize energy expenditure per unit distance. When moving at slower or faster speeds, more energy is required (Mochon and McMahon 1980; Shumway-Cook et al. 2023c). Therefore, gait speed at one's preferred pace may be the most meaningful measure.

Distances for testing gait velocity also vary, with common lengths being 10 m or 4 m. The 10-m walk test (10 mWT) is the most frequently used (Menezes-Oliveira et al. 2021; Collen et al. 1990). As gait velocity stabilizes after about 3 steps, many tests incorporate extra distance to eliminate the acceleration (e.g., 2 m) and deceleration phases (e.g., 2 m) of gait (Menezes-Oliveira et al. 2021).

Gait velocity is usually measured using a stopwatch, although other measurement tools like a radar can also be employed.

Different test numbers are utilized, with measuring the same distance three times and averaging the three scores being a common approach.

Since walking velocity can be influenced by age and gender, gender- and age-specific normal values have been reported (Bohannon 1997). In young adults, for example, walking at about 1.46 m/s (3.26 miles/h) has been found to be common (Shumway-Cook et al. 2023a; Craik 1989). A velocity of 1.4 m/s is considered the minimum speed required to safely cross a street.

5.4.2 Timed Up and Go Test

In daily life, mobility includes standing up, sitting down, initiating walking, continuous walking, and changing walking direction. The Timed Up and Go (TUG) test is a simple assessment of functional mobility (Menezes-Oliveira et al. 2021). Originally, the Get Up and Go test was developed to screen for balance problems in older adults (Mathias et al. 1986), but it was later modified by incorporating a timed component (Podsiadlo and Richardson 1991), such as by establishing age-specific normal values for the 3 meter test in healthy women (Isles et al. 2004). Additionally, age and gender-specific normal values for the 8-foot test in the elderly were reported (Rikli and Jones 2001). To enhance the sensitivity and specificity of fall risk assessment, a dual-task TUG incorporating a cognitive task was developed (Shumway-Cook et al. 2000). The advantage of this test lies in its simplicity, quick administration time, and validity for evaluating functional mobility levels and fall risk among older adults living in a community.

5.4.3 Step Length

Step length refers to the distance from one foot's initial contact to the following foot's initial contact. Step length can be used to assess gait asymmetry. In young adults, for instance, the average step length has been found to be 76.3 cm (Shumway-Cook et al. 2023a; Craik 1989).

5.4.4 Stride Length

Stride length, on the other hand, is the distance from one foot's initial contact to the subsequent contact of the same foot.

5.4.5 Step Frequency/Cadence

Cadence represents the number of steps taken within a specified unit of time, often reported as steps per minute. Sometimes, cadence can be expressed as the number of strides per unit of time, which is denoted as strides per minute. In normal adults walking at a self-selected speed, the step count typically averages around 110 and 115 steps per minute for males and females, respectively (Finley and Cody 1970; Murray et al. 1984, SC 16).

5.4.6 Step Width

Step width signifies the horizontal distance between the center of the heel markers of one foot and the subsequent foot. An increased step width is observed in individuals with poor balance, such as those with cerebellar ataxia. Older adults with a history of falls tend to exhibit greater step width compared to those without such a history (Heitmann et al. 1989).

5.4.7 Endurance

Considering that community ambulation necessitates not only speed but also endurance, measuring the distance an individual can walk within a specified time frame is crucial. Many individuals with chronic stroke have reported that the ability to walk longer distances is vital for engaging in both home and community activities (Combs et al. 2013). Although the 2-min, 3-min, and 6-min walk tests are less sensitive than the 12-min walk test, they offer reliable results (Butland et al. 1982). The 6-min walk test is considered one of the best predictors of community ambulation (Fulk et al. 2017), with age- and gender-specific normative values for the 6-min walk test having already been established (Rikli and Jones 2001). In order to increase walking distance, improvements in endurance and a reduction in the energy cost of walking are necessary factors that must be addressed.

5.5 Assessment Using Gait Pattern (Kinematics)

5.5.1 Observational Gait Analysis

Observational gait analysis is the most commonly used method for gait assessment as it requires no special equipment, making it exceptionally convenient. Observation is typically carried out from the back and side of the individual walking. Video recordings can also aid in observational gait analysis. Nevertheless, this method has several limitations, including the time required to acquire the proper observational skills, its generally poor reliability, the inherent difficulty in observing transverse plane movements, and limited sensitivity in detecting changes in gait patterns (Krebs et al. 1985). That said, the use of standardized forms can assist in systematic evaluation and documentation (Winter 1993). The Rancho Los Amigos Gait Analysis Form documents gait patterns according to the phases of the gait cycle (Los Amigos Research and Education Institute 1989).

Three-dimensional trajectory of the CoM motion assumes a figure-eight shape and may be a promising summary index of both balance and the neural maturation of walking (Tesio and Rota 2019).

5.5.2 Optoelectric Analysis System

The optoelectric analysis system employs 6–10 cameras and markers to assess three-dimensional body motion during walking. It is highly sensitive, reliable at detecting gait patterns, and considered the gold standard for gait pattern assessment. However, this system does have limitations, which include its high cost, space and technical expertise requirements, and high time consumption.

5.5.3 Systems Using Motion Sensors

Motion sensors are highly sensitive to detecting body segment movements and are becoming more affordable. However, commercially available equipment remains somewhat expensive. If costs become more accessible, this technology could greatly assist in gait assessment.

5.5.4 Smartphone Apps

Nowadays, AI programs have been developed to assess human motion using multiple smartphone cameras, eliminating the need for markers. These programs provide three-dimensional data regarding human motion. With the continued development of this technology, it may become possible to conveniently assess gait patterns at a lower cost.

5.6 Assessment Using Kinetics

Motion analysis systems and force plates can be used to assess the kinetics of individual joints. While these systems have limitations, such as their high cost, time consumption, and space and technical expertise requirements, they offer valuable information including gait regularity, asymmetry, trajectory of the center of mass, and joint power. Kinetic parameters such as paretic propulsion power have been recommended as primary outcome measures for post-stroke gait rehabilitation (Roelker et al. 2019). However, until these systems are no longer bound by their limitations, they will not be practical in clinical applications.

5.7 Summary

Gait assessment can be performed through a variety of approaches, including subjective tests, disability level assessments, quantitative tests, and gait pattern analyses. To capture the full spectrum of an individual's gait, a combination of tests from different perspectives is necessary.

Quantitative evaluation is essential to confirm the effectiveness of walking training. Gait velocity is one of the most commonly used tests to evaluate gait function, and it is considered the single best measure due to its simplicity, reliability, and lack of time constraints.

Observational gait analysis is the most commonly used method to evaluate gait pattern, but it has several limitations, including the time required to acquire skill, poor reliability, difficulty in observing transverse plane movements, and limited sensitivity in detecting changes in gait patterns. However, the future is promising as newly developed technologies could solve these problems.

References

Andrews AW. Self-report measures of mobility. Top Geriatr Rehabil. 2012;28(1):2–10.

Bohannon RW. Comfortable and maximum walking speed of adults aged 20–79 years: reference values and determinants. Age Ageing. 1997;26(1):15–9.

Brandstater ME, de Bruin H, Gowland C, Clark BM. Hemiplegic gait: analysis of temporal variables. Arch Phys Med Rehabil. 1983;64(12):583–7.

Butland RJ, Pang J, Gross ER, Woodcock AA, Geddes DM. Two-, six-, and 12-min walking tests in respiratory disease. Br Med J (Clin Res Ed). 1982;284(6329):1607–8.

Collen FM, Wade DT, Bradshaw CM. Mobility after stroke: reliability of measures of impairment and disability. Int Disabil Stud. 1990;12(1):6–9.

Combs SA, Van Puymbroeck M, Altenburger PA, Miller KK, Dierks TA, Schmid AA. Is walking faster or walking farther more important to persons with chronic stroke? Disabil Rehabil. 2013;35:860–7.

Craik R. Changes in locomotor in the aging adult. In: Woollacott MH, Shumway-Cook A, editors. Development of posture and gait: across the life span. Columbia: University of South Carolina; 1989. p. 176–201.

Cyarto EV, Myers AM, Tudor-Locke C. Pedometer accuracy in nursing home and community-dwelling older adults. Med Sci Sports Exerc. 2004;36(2):205–9.

Farin E, Fleitz A, Frey C. Psychometric properties of an International Classification of Functioning, Disability and Health (ICF)-oriented, adaptive questionnaire for the assessment of mobility, self-care and domestic life. J Rehabil Med. 2007;39(7):537–46.

Finley FR, Cody KA. Locomotive characteristics of urban pedestrians. Arch Phys Med Rehabil. 1970;51(7):423–6.

Fulk GD, He Y, Boyne P, Dunning K. Predicting home and community walking activity poststroke. Stroke. 2017;48(2):406–11. https://doi.org/10.1016/j.apmr.2005.09.014.

Gray DB, Hollingsworth HH, Stark SL, Morgan KA. Participation survey/mobility: psychometric properties of a measure of participation for people with mobility impairments and limitations. Arch Phys Med Rehabil. 2006;87(2):189–97.

Heitmann DK, Gossman MR, Shaddeau SA, Jackson JR. Balance performance and step width in noninstitutionalized, elderly, female fallers and nonfallers. Phys Ther. 1989;69(11):923–31.

Isles RC, Choy NLL, Steer M, Nitz JC. Normal values of balance tests in women aged 20–80. J Am Geriatr Soc. 2004;52(8):1367–72.

Krebs DE, Edelstein JE, Fishman S. Reliability of observational kinematic gait analysis. Phys Ther. 1985;65(7):1027–33.

Lord SE, McPherson K, McNaughton HK, Rochester L, Weatherall M. Community ambulation after stroke: how important and obtainable is it and what measures appear predictive? Arch Phys Med Rehabil. 2004;85(2):234–9.

Los Amigos Research and Education Institute. Observational gait analysis handbook. Downey: Los Amigos Research and Education Institute, Rancho Los Amigos Medical Center; 1989. p. 55.

Mathias S, Nayak US, Isaacs B. Balance in elderly patients: the "get-up and go" test. Arch Phys Med Rehabil. 1986;67(6):387–9.

Menezes-Oliveira E, Matuti GDS, de Oliveira CB, de Freitas SF, Kawamura CM, Lopes JAF, Arida RM. Effects of lower extremity constraint-induced movement therapy on gait and balance of chronic hemiparetic patients after stroke: description of a study protocol for a randomized controlled clinical trial. Trials. 2021;22:463.

Mochon S, McMahon TA. Ballistic walking. J Biomech. 1980;13(1):49–57.

Murray MP, Kory RC, Sepic SB. Walking patterns of normal women. Arch Phys Med Rehabil. 1970;51(11):637–50.

Murray MP, Mollinger LA, Gardner GM, Sepic SB. Kinematic and EMG patterns during slow, free, and fast walking. J Orthop Res. 1984;2(3):272–80.

Perry J, Garrett M, Gronley JK, Mulroy SJ. Classification of walking handicap in the stroke population. Stroke. 1995;26(6):982–9.

Podsiadlo D, Richardson S. The timed "Up & Go": a test of basic functional mobility for frail elderly persons. J Am Geriatr Soc. 1991;39(2):142–8.

Richards CI. Gait velocity as an outcome measure of locomotor recovery after stroke. In: Craik RL, Oatis CS, editors. Gait analysis: theory and application. St. Louis: Mosby; 1995. p. 355–64.

Rikli RE, Jones CJ. Senior fitness test manual. Champaign: Human Kinetics; 2001.

Roelker SA, Bowden MG, Kautz SA, Neptune RR. Paretic propulsion as a measure of walking performance and functional motor recovery post-stroke: a review. Gait Posture. 2019;68:6–14.

Shumway-Cook A, Brauer S, Woollacott M. Predicting the probability for falls in community-dwelling older adults using the Timed Up & Go Test. Phys Ther. 2000;80(9):896–903.

Shumway-Cook A, Woollacott MH, Rachwani J, Santamaria V. Control of normal mobility (Chapter 12). In: Motor control: translating research into clinical practice. 6th ed. Philadelphia: Lippincott Williams & Wilkins; 2023a. p. 333–66.

Shumway-Cook A, Woollacott MH, Rachwani J, Santamaria V. Aging and mobility (Chapter 14). In: Motor control: translating research into clinical practice. 6th ed. Philadelphia: Lippincott Williams & Wilkins; 2023b. p. 389–406.

Shumway-Cook A, Woollacott MH, Rachwani J, Santamaria V. Clinical management of the patient with a mobility disorder (Chapter 16). In: Motor control: translating research into clinical practice. 6th ed. Philadelphia: Lippincott Williams & Wilkins; 2023c. p. 440–89.

Tesio L, Rota V. The motion of body center of mass during walking: a review oriented to clinical applications. Front Neurol. 2019;10:999.

Viosca E, Martínez JL, Almagro PL, Gracia A, González C. Proposal and validation of a new functional ambulation classification scale for clinical use. Arch Phys Med Rehabil. 2005;86(6):1234–8.

Wade DT. Measurement in neurological rehabilitation. Oxford: Oxford Medical Publications; 1992.

Wendel N, Macpherson CE, Webber K, Hendron K, DeAngelis T, Colon-Semenza C, Ellis T. Accuracy of activity trackers in Parkinson disease: should we prescribe them? Phys Ther. 2018;98(8):705–14.

Winter DA. Knowledge base for diagnostic gait assessments. Med Progr Technol. 1993;19(2):61–81.

Assessment of Muscle Strength 6

6.1 Overview of Muscle Strength Test

6.1.1 Importance of Muscle Strength

Muscle strength is not only essential for performing daily activities but also serves as an important predictor of the length of hospital stays, hospital readmission rates, mortality as it relates to mobility, and unfavorable outcomes (Bohannon 2019).

6.1.2 Purpose of Muscle Strength Test

The muscle strength test is used to identify weakness and detect changes in muscle strength. It is difficult to detect changes in muscle strength without the use of a quantitative test.

6.1.3 Proper Test of Muscle Strength

A proper test requires the use of standardized procedures and a well-trained tester. If it is impossible to test muscle strength in a standardized position, it is essential to note that test has been performed out of the recommended protocol.

Standardized procedures should provide protocol for adequate stabilization (Bohannon 2019), postural stability, and familiarization of people with gait disability to strength test.

Providing postural stability is of utmost importance while taking a strength test, and it can be achieved by simply resting a hand on the wall (Hébert-Losier et al. 2017).

Muscle strength can be tested using one repetition maximum (maximal contraction) or multiple repetition maximum (submaximal contraction).

To test a subject's one-repetition maximum, the muscle should be contracted to its maximum ability, and it should be a voluntary contraction (Bohannon 2019).

A strength test with a handheld dynamometer can be used to evaluate a subject's one-repetition maximum.

Since submaximal contractions are safer to perform for patients and the elderly than maximal contractions, many functional tests, such as the sit-to-stand test, make use of submaximal contractions.

If possible, tests should be completed at the same time of the day.

6.1.4 Field Tests

Field tests refer to tests that are used in clinical environments, community settings, or home settings (Regterschot et al. 2015).

To be a field test, it must first be practical. Many factors are involved when assessing the

Y.-S. Lee, *Task Oriented Gait Training*, https://doi.org/10.1007/978-981-97-3348-4_6

practicality, including the cost of equipment, the space required by the equipment, the portability of the equipment, safety (risk of injury), the duration of the measurement, and the ease of data acquisition.

Since there is no test that is completely reliable, valid, and practical, further development of tests is necessary.

The manual muscle test, handheld dynamometry, and functional tests (e.g., the sit-to-stand test, the "heel raise" test, etc.) can be used as field tests.

6.2 Manual Muscle Test

6.2.1 Overview of the Manual Muscle Test

The manual muscle test is a test performed using gravity or the application of an external load by the tester. It does not require any additional equipment and the test can be performed quickly (Pfister et al. 2018). In addition, it can be used to assess almost any muscle of body. Therefore, the manual muscle test is the current standard.

6.2.1.1 Types of Muscle Contractions

The manual muscle test is performed using voluntary muscle contraction. If spontaneous muscle contraction is used in people unable to cooperate well, this must be noted clearly.

6.2.1.2 Use of Qualitative Terms

Previously, results of manual muscle tests were recorded with the use of qualitative terms, such as zero, poor, fair, good, or normal. However, it is not recommended that the tester utilize such qualitative terms, as in some muscles, as low as 10% of normal muscle strength can be classified as "good."

6.2.1.3 Modes of Test

Manual muscle tests can be performed either through "make tests" or "break tests." In a make test, people perform the full range of joint motion against maximal resistance. And in a break test, people must maintain a position against maximal resistance (load). Because it is more difficult to do a make test, break tests are more widely used.

6.2.2 Grading of Muscle Strength

6.2.2.1 Muscle Strength Grade 1

The observation of muscle contraction or the feeling of muscle contraction is used for muscle grade 1.

This may be an objective or subjective test. However, to be useful, muscle contraction should be selective.

In some people with upper motor neuron lesions, muscle contraction is not selective. In such cases, the context should be described clearly. Also, the frequent induction of nonselective muscle contractions may be harmful to functional recovery.

Since it is impossible to observe or palpate deep muscle, grade 1 cannot be used to evaluate deep muscles.

6.2.2.2 Muscle Strength Grade 2

To minimize the effect of gravity, tests for grade 2 muscles are usually done in a side-lying position.

Muscle strength grade 2 is considered a critical grade because muscles that are assigned grade 2 can easily be strengthened with voluntary muscle contractions. Muscles classified as grade 1 can also be strengthened through a voluntary contraction, but it is more difficulty to do so.

Voluntary movement can be facilitated by posture and joint alignment. If voluntary joint movement cannot be observed, a change in posture and joint alignment may be helpful.

Placing the hip in a slightly flexed position with manual assistance can help hip flexion in people who show no voluntary joint motion in a fully extended hip position (Fig. 6.1). This means that slight hip flexion can make hip flexion more easily achievable.

Grade 2 minus can be assigned when there is intermittent voluntary motion or when voluntary movement is only possible when facilitation is provided (e.g., bilateral co-contraction of hip adduction).

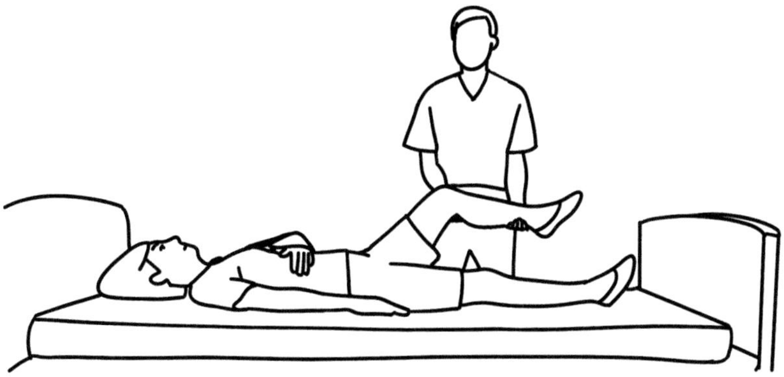

Fig. 6.1 Test of hip flexors with partial hip flexion in a supine position. Sightly assisting hip flexion using manual assistance can help achieve hip flexion in people who show no voluntary joint motion in a fully extended hip position

Grade 2 plus is a strength classification in which a subject can move the joint voluntarily against gravity but only within less than half of the range of motion (Brown and Avers 2018a).

6.2.2.3 Muscle Strength Grade 3

Grade 3 can be assigned when there is a full range of motion that can voluntarily be made against gravity. If the range of motion is incomplete, grade 3 minus can be given (Brown and Avers 2018a).

If people require compensation to complete the full range of motion (such as using a posterior lean of the trunk to facilitate knee extension), grade 3 minus can be given.

6.2.2.4 Muscle Strength Grade 4

To assign grade 4, there must be a full active range of motion observed against gravity. After this, it must be possible for the subject to hold this joint position against gravity and submaximal resistance.

Muscle grade 4 in a manual muscle test is subjective, and the range of acceptance is very wide. In some muscles, 10% of normal muscle strength can be classified as muscle grade 4 (Dvir 1997).

Therefore, there is no sensitivity when detecting a change of muscle strength.

6.2.2.5 Muscle Strength Grade 5

To be classified as grade 5, there must be a full active range of motion against gravity. After performing this full range of motion, the subject must be capable of maintaining this position against gravity and maximal resistance (external load).

Manual muscle tests of grade 5 muscles are subjective in nature. This is partially due to the fact that it is difficult for a tester to apply maximal resistance without having strong muscle strength themselves.

To apply maximal resistance, gravity, body weight, and the use of the longest lever arm are required. To apply maximal resistance using gravity, the direction of manual resistance must be applied downward vertically. By placing the hand of the tester at the more distant part of a limb from the axis of rotation, it is possible to apply more resistance.

In ankle plantar flexor, manual resistance is inadequate to apply maximal resistance to the muscle. If the test of ankle plantar flexor is done with manual resistance in a supine position, there is a high probability of overestimation of strength. To solve this problem, many other tests, such as the heel lift test and test using isokinetic dynamometer, are being developed and used.

In a manual muscle test, the maximal voluntary contraction is used, with the exception of the ankle plantar flexor. Since it is difficult to apply maximal resistance (load) to the ankle plantar flexor using only the body weight of the subject, a number of full heel lifts using a single limb is necessary.

One important thing to consider is that classification should be done in order to compare with young healthy people, likewise T score in bond densitometry (Brown and Avers 2018a). As the weakness in elderly subjects leads to functional disability, elderly people can increase muscle strength with strength training. When classifying muscle strength in elderly people, people with weak muscles may still be classified as grade 5. However, if muscle strength is classified grade 5, it leads to a loss of opportunity to increase muscle strength (Brown and Avers 2018a).

6.2.3 Limitations of the Manual Muscle Test

The manual muscle test requires that the tester have adequate muscle strength to apply maximal resistance. If the tester does not possess adequate strength, the results of the test may become unreliable. In addition, it is physically demanding to the tester. As such, tests for grades 4 and 5 are subjective tests, which implies that they have limited reliability (Bohannon 2019).

It is difficult to detect changes of muscle strength over time (due to poor sensitivity) (Pfister et al. 2018; Bohannon 2019).

The range of grade 4 is extremely broad, so many test results lead to a classification of grade 4 despite there being an actual change in muscle strength. To check whether there is actual change of muscle strength, a quantitative test is required. And the manual muscle test has a ceiling effect (Bohannon 2019). In addition to this, it lacks normative values (Pfister et al. 2018).

6.3 Tests Using Closed Kinetic Chain Muscle Contraction

Tests using closed kinetic chain muscle contraction have several advantages. Firstly, they can test several muscles simultaneously, and they have more similar biomechanics to real-life muscle use.

Omnikinetic machines use closed kinetic muscle contraction and inverse dynamics. These machines can provide power and net joint torque (Davis and Dolny 2000). Although they provide useful information, these machines are not used widely due to their high cost, space requirements, and general inconvenience (time setup analysis).

6.3.1 Heel Lift

It is extremely difficult to test the muscle strength of the ankle plantar using an external load applied by a tester as it is a strong muscle and has a short lever arm. Testing through the use of manual resistance assesses only 18% of a person's ability to do a single, complete heel rise (Beasley 1961).

Therefore, in many protocols of manual muscle tests, the ankle plantar flexor is tested using body weight instead of manual resistance. To provide postural stability, having the subject rest their hands on the wall can be helpful (Hébert-Losier et al. 2017). To be classified as grade 3, a muscle must be able to move the subject's body weight in a full range of motion at the ankle joint. However, the range of motion of the ankle joint is not the same in all people, especially in those with a gait disability (Fig. 6.2).

Performing a heel lift with both lower extremities while in a standing position is one possible

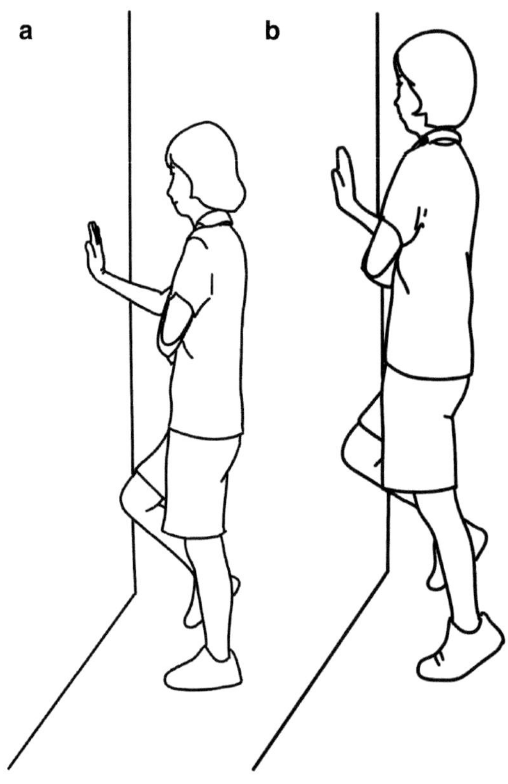

Fig. 6.2 Heel lift: (**a**) starting position of heel lift; (**b**) final position of heel lift

method to check the range of motion of the ankle joint. However, this method has its own limitations since many elderly people cannot lift their heels fully even when using both lower extremities.

If people cannot reach the full range of motion with one lower extremity, the muscle strength must be classified as less than grade 3.

To be classified as grade 5, it should be possible for the subject to perform a full range of motion heel lift for 20 consecutive repetitions.

Since many elderly people and people with gait disabilities cannot achieve full range with one lower extremity, testing the ankle plantar flexor is extremely important.

The heel lift test has many advantages. Not only is it reliable, but it does not require any equipment, and there is no physical burden on the tester and no need for time to set up or process the data.

6.3.2 Sit-to-Stand Test

The sit-to-stand test is a very useful test to assess muscle strength in a lower extremity. It is easy to perform as there is no need for the tester to provide resistance, and it does not require any expensive equipment. In addition, the results of the test are objective and provide a continuous data.

Since this test uses body weight as its load, there is no need to apply an external load, and the test results do not depend on the strength of the examiner (Fig. 6.3).

If a subject cannot move their center of mass forward, they cannot perform a sit-to-stand test even if they have adequate muscle strength. In such a situation, pushing the trunk forward may be helpful in assisting people to stand by themselves.

To perform the sit-to-stand test easily, 15° of ankle dorsiflexion is required (Carr and Shepherd 2010). Ankle contracture may prevent ankle dorsiflexion and interfere forward movement of the center of mass. In such a case, it is helpful to perform a sit-to-stand test by placing flat material under the subject's heels.

In addition, the height of the chair used in a sit-to-stand test can be adjusted according to the height of the subject (from 30 to 60 cm), or it may be fixed (as in with a standard chair).

The sit-to-stand test using both lower extremities is assessed according to two methods.

The first makes use of the number of sit-to-stand performed in a predetermined time. Thirty seconds is the most frequently used duration, and it is often used in senior fitness tests. At other times, 15-s or 1-min durations may be used.

Another method utilizes the time to complete a predetermined number of sit-to-stand. The "5 Times Chair Rise Test" is most frequently used in Short Physical Performance Battery. Other repetition numbers, such as one time or ten times, can be used.

Tests using the sit-to-stand using both lower extremities have several limitations.

First of all, it is not purely a strength test (Whitney et al. 2005) as it can be affected by balance capacity (Lord et al. 2002; McCarthy et al. 2004). In people with stroke, performance on the five-time STS was correlated with balance (BBS) but not muscle strength (Ng 2010).

Since touching the wall with both hands during a sit-to-stand test can decrease the balance requirement, it may be helpful to make a sit-to-stand test that relies more on pure muscle strength.

Secondly, it is difficult to test people with asymmetric weakness. The sit-to-stand test is usually done using both lower extremities, so the results are a sum of the strength of both legs. The result of a sit-to-stand test does not provide useful information regarding muscle strength of an individual lower extremity. In this case, a one-legged sit-to-stand test may prove useful for people with asymmetric lower extremity weakness (Thongchoomsin et al. 2020).

The third thing to consider is that this test has a floor effect, which means that it may be too difficult for people with severe muscle weakness to complete. For example, it would be impossible to use the "5 Times Chair Rise Test" to test people who cannot complete a sit-to-stand five times due to severe muscle weakness.

Lastly, the result of this test is affected by the height of the subject. If a standard chair is used for people of varying heights, it may be easy for

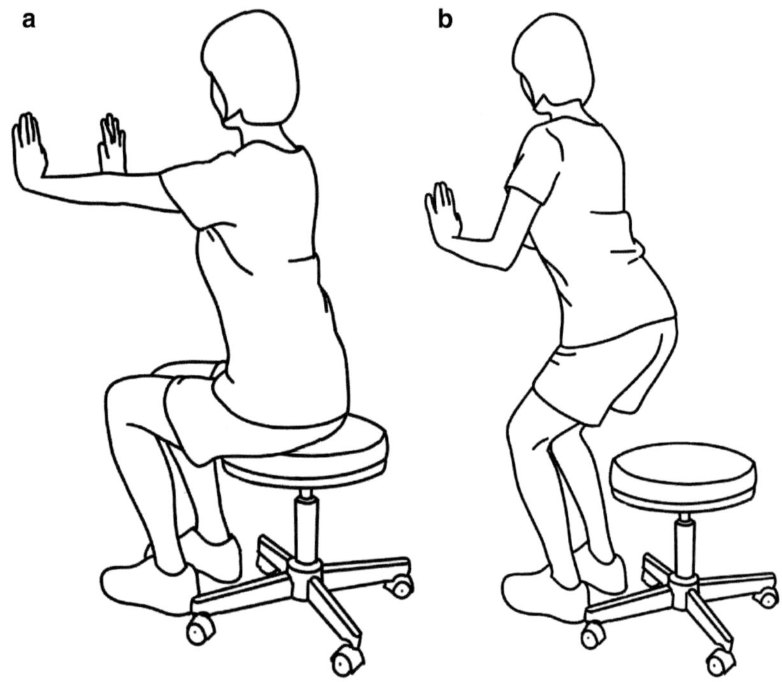

Fig. 6.3 Sit-to-stand test with wall touch: (**a**) starting position of sit-to-stand test; (**b**) midpoint of sit-to-stand test

shorter people to complete the sit-to-stand test; however, it may prove difficult for taller people.

6.3.3 Bridging

Bridging can be used as a screening test to verify whether a subject suffers from lower extremity muscle weakness. As it can be performed in a supine position, it is very useful for people who have difficulty getting out of bed due to mobility problem.

To perform bridging with one lower limb, first flex the hip and knee joint of the testing leg, and then place the foot on the floor. Following this, lift the contralateral lower limb while maintaining knee joint extension. Finally, lift the hip as high as possible using the ipsilateral lower limb (Fig. 6.4).

Many muscles of the body are involved in bridging, such as the hip extensor, knee flexor, and trunk extensor. Bridging with one lower limb can be used to check the weakness of lower extremity muscles. If people cannot lift their buttocks fully off the floor using only one lower extremity, this suggests weakness of that extremity. If there is moderate weakness in one leg, the height of hip lift or the speed of hip lift will be less than what is observed on the contralateral side. If there is more severe weakness, it may be impossible to lift hip at all.

In addition, bridging can be useful in detecting paresis of the lower limb in people with hemiparesis. If hemiparesis is present, when bridging, the performance of the affected lower limb will prove to be different from that of the other limb. Strength can be assessed using the height at which the subject is able to lift the buttocks: full, partial, minimal, not at all.

Other information, such as obliquity of the pelvis and the need for external support when bridging, is useful to record. If there is weakness in the hip internal rotator, this may cause obliquity of the pelvis. If there is weakness in the knee flexor, the foot may slide down and need to be held foot by tester.

Bridging with both lower extremities can be used to check the possibility of standing transfer in bed-ridden patients. If people can lift their buttocks with both lower extremities, they may have the ability to support their body weight (totally or partially). In that case, a standing transfer can be tried with the assistance of other people.

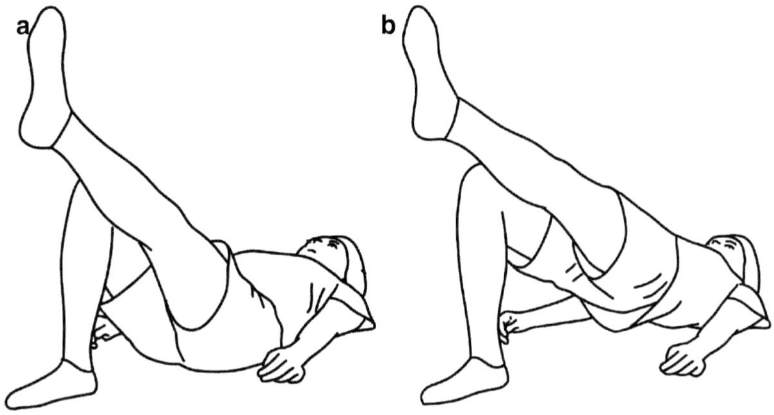

Fig. 6.4 Bridging with one leg: (**a**) starting position of bridging with one leg; (**b**) final position of bridging with one leg

Despite its usefulness, bridging has several limitations. One is the ceiling effect. People with mild weakness may still manage to lift their buttocks in the full range of motion using one lower extremity. Second is the difficulty in quantifying the data resulting from the test. It is difficult to measure the amount that the buttocks lift, for example. So, it may be helpful to use a pressure sensor under the foot.

Third, this test is difficult to perform for people with hip flexion contracture.

Still, it may be possible to quantify the strength of a lower extremity using ground reaction force (Eliassen et al. 2018) as the change of ground reaction force depends on the amount of muscle contraction (and the height to which the buttocks can lift).

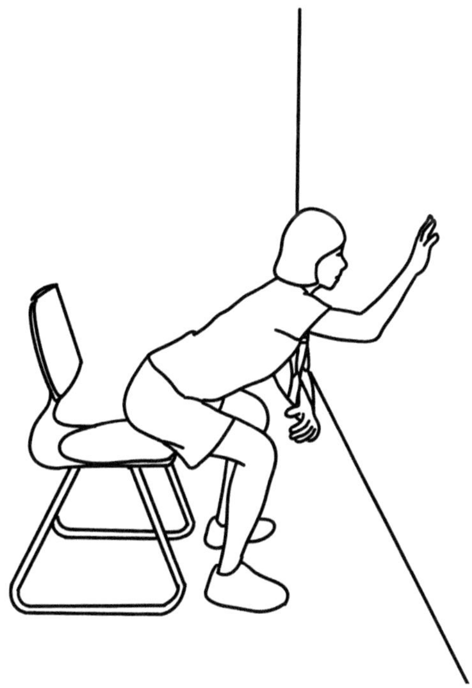

Fig. 6.5 Squat with chair

6.3.4 Squat Using Both Lower Limbs

Squats are commonly used to strengthen lower extremity muscles, but they can also be used to test the muscle strength of the lower extremities. The squat test using both lower limbs is carried out in the following manner.

First, the subject must stand on two legs while facing the wall. A chair will be placed behind them. The subject must then raise their arms and touch the wall and flex their legs so that their hips touch the seat of the chair. After this, they must go back to the starting position (Fig. 6.5). This same action should be repeated until the specified number of times or duration has been reached. The difference from the sit-to-stand test is that it starts in a standing position, and the hips only touch the seat; the subject should never sit fully in the chair.

A hand on the wall provides posture stability, and the chair prevents people from falling down and getting injured.

The limitation of the squat test using both lower limbs is that it is difficult to evaluate the asymmetric weakness of the lower limbs.

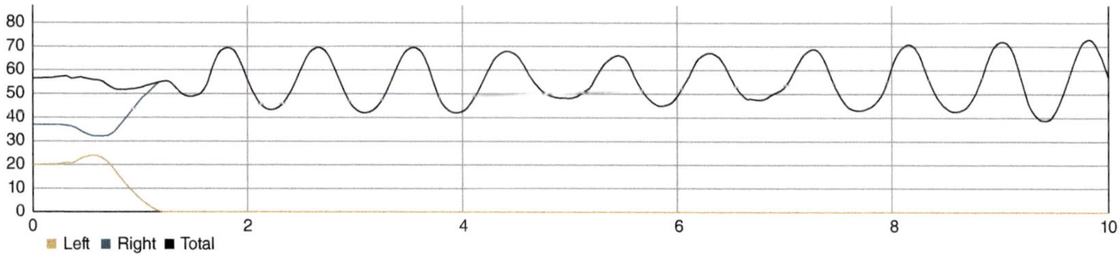

Fig. 6.6 Change of ground reaction force during squat test using one lower limb

6.3.5 Squat Test Using One Lower Limb

The squat test can be done using a single lower limb to evaluate the muscle strength of an individual lower limb. A single-leg squat test is often used to assess movement quality, balance, stability, knee control, overall motor control, and dynamic alignment of the body (Lewis et al. 2015).

The advantage of a single-leg squat is that it is convenient (Zawadka et al. 2020); however, this test has several limitations. For example, the number of repetitions that should be aimed for is affected by the height of the subject.

It may be possible to quantify the amount of contraction of extensor muscles of the lower limb as it correlates with movement of the center of mass using ground reaction force (Eliassen et al. 2018). Changes in the ground reaction force depend on the amount of lower extremity flexion and extension. Figure 6.6 shows the change of ground reaction force during multiple repetitions of squatting using a single lower limb.

6.4 Dynamometer

6.4.1 Overview

Since a quantitative value is essential to detect changes in muscle strength, the quantitative testing of muscle strength has a long history. For instance, in 1915, the quantitative assessment of muscle strength using a sling spring scale was reported (Martin and Lovett 1915).

Quantitative muscle strength tests are usually performed with a dynamometer. This tool provides an objective test result and provides continuous data. In addition, this tool is sufficiently sensitive to reliably check changes in muscle strength.

Dynamometers are used primarily in research, and usage in the field is limited these days due to a variety of reasons.

6.4.2 Handheld Dynamometer

A handheld dynamometer is useful and has many advantages. Firstly, it can provide quantitative values of peak force expressed in Newtons. It also has proven validity (Stark et al. 2011) and reliability (Pfister et al. 2018). In addition, it can be used with a variety of muscles. Since its size is compact, it is also portable, its cost is not restrictive, and it is easy to use.

The muscle strength test using handheld dynamometer by applying make method has better agreement and less rater-dependence than break method (González-Rosalén et al. 2021).

One limitation is that a dynamometer requires the strength of the tester to maintain the position of the dynamometer. To solve this problem, diverse methods are employed, such as the use of steel frames, polyethylene tubes, and bands.

6.4.3 Isokinetic Dynamometer

Tests using an isokinetic dynamometer are recognized as being the gold standard of strength tests (Jackson et al. 2017). An isokinetic dynamometer allows for the reliable testing of concentric, eccentric, and isometric muscle contractions (Kristensen et al. 2017).

Isokinetic dynamometers consist of a large steel frame, a motorized component that provides controlled motion, and a dynamometer.

While they are reliable, tests using an isokinetic machine have many limitations. For example, the equipment is prohibitively expensive. They are also heavy and lack portability as they are large and require adequate space. These machines also require the tester to have proper training and expertise. Also, since the body moves in an isotonic manner, not isokinetic, it does not accurately match movement in the real world. Lastly, the time needed to conduct a test using the equipment is prohibitively long, so it is not practical in most clinical situations.

6.4.4 Traction Dynamometer

A traction dynamometer can be fixed to a solid object more easily than a handheld dynamometer. Also, there are many traction dynamometers available on the commercial market. Since they are not expensive and are easy to use, these tools may be useful when a quantitative test of muscle strength is required.

6.5 Force Plate

A force plate is used to test muscle strength in research. While performing a unilateral squat, it is possible to evaluate peak vertical ground reaction force and the rate of force development using a force plate (Eliassen et al. 2018).

6.6 Sliding Tilt Table

A sliding tilt table consists of a supporting frame, tilting frame, sliding top, motor to change the inclination angle of the tilting frame, friction-reducing mechanism, leg raiser, goniometer, and device for changing the range of motion (Fig. 6.7).

This machine is similar to the leg press machines commonly found in gyms. It provides minimized friction and makes it possible to exercise in a gravity-controlled condition through the inclination of its tilting frame.

Since external load is increased with the inclination angle of a tilting frame, this machine can

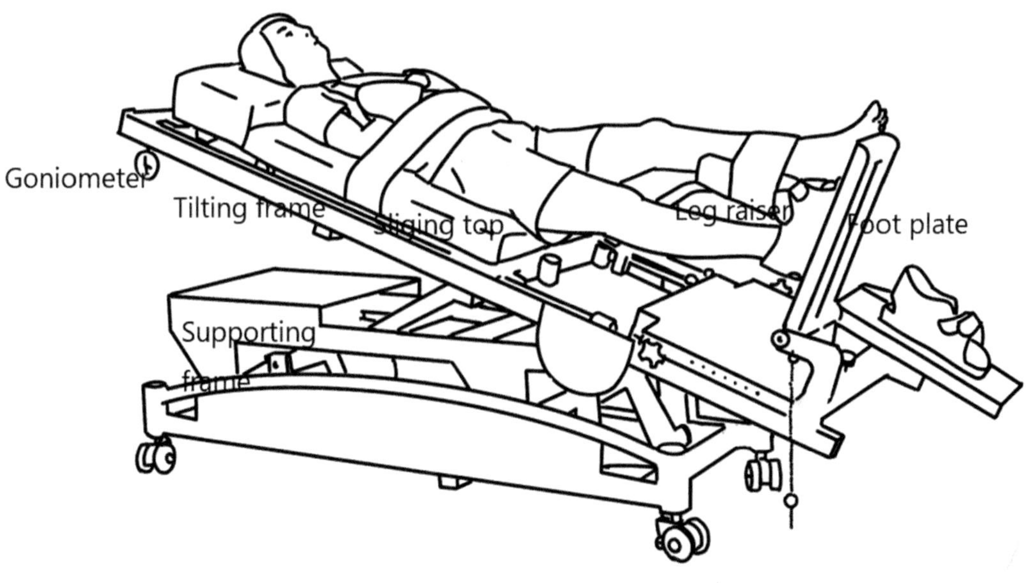

Fig. 6.7 Sliding tilt table

be used to test the muscle strength of the lower extremities. It is also useful for checking changes in muscle strength. At a particular angle, the repetition number is determined by muscle strength. Information regarding the angle and repetition number is easy to record, and this data may be helpful for improving the motivation of people with a gait disability.

6.7 Test of Individual Muscles

6.7.1 Spinal (Back) Extensor

Since many people who use walking aids demonstrate a weakness of the spinal extensor, this weakness can be implicated in their gait. Thus, a test of the spinal extensor is critical in people with a gait disability.

Spinal extensors can be classified into lumbar spine extensors and thoracic spine extensors. To perform a test of the lumbar extensor, people must lie down in a prone position with their fingers touching the side of the head, and their shoulders in external rotation. The examiner should stabilize the subject's lower extremities just above the ankles. To achieve a level of grade 5, the subject must be able to raise their head, shoulders, and chest to the end position quickly and hold that position without evidence of significant effort. To perform a test of the thoracic spine extensor, the subject must lie down in a prone position, with their head and upper trunk extending off the table from about the nipple. In addition, their fingers should be touching the side of the head, and their shoulders and elbows must be retracted. The examiner needs to stabilize the subject's lower extremities just above the ankles. To achieve a level of grade 5, the subject must be able to raise the upper trunk quickly from its forward flexed position to the horizontal position with ease and no sign of exertion (Brown and Avers 2018b).

To achieve a grade 3, the subject must take a prone position with their arms at their sides. They must then lift their head, shoulders, chest, and umbilicus enough to clear the table (Brown and Avers 2018b).

It should be noted that tests of the spinal extensor in the prone position are somewhat inconvenient in outpatient clinics. Back extensor strength can be tested in a sitting position more conveniently. Reaching forward in a sitting position while maintaining back extension or picking up object on the floor may be used as a screening test for back extension weakness (Fig. 6.8).

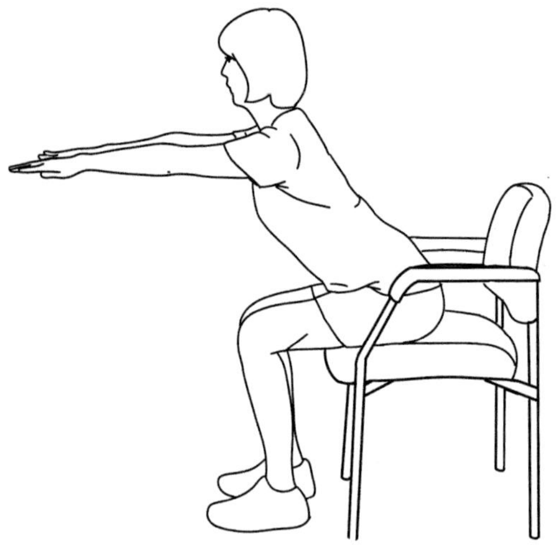

Fig. 6.8 Reaching forward with hands in the air

6.7.2 Hip Internal Rotator

If there is asymmetry in the hip external rotation between the two lower limbs in a supine or sitting position, this suggests a weakness of the hip internal rotator in the more external rotated lower limb.

When testing the hip flexor in a supine position or sitting position, if external rotation of hip occurs, this is an indicator that there is weakness of the internal rotator.

If there is external rotation of the hip during bridging, this suggests weakness of the hip internal rotator in that limb.

6.7.3 Hip Flexor

6.7.3.1 Grade 2

For people who are bed-ridden and constantly in a supine position, testing in a supine position with full hip extension may be more convenient than testing with the subject in a side-lying position. If there is no hip flexion observed in a supine position, changing starting position from full hip extension to slight hip flexion may help with hip flexion. If the subject is able to flex their hip fully, it may be possible to test the subject in a sitting position. If the subject is unable to flex their hip in a supine position, there is no choice but to test the subject in a side-lying position. If the subject can flex their hip joint in a side-lying position, their muscle grade is considered grade 2.

6.7.3.2 Grade 3

In a sitting position, the patient can complete the full range of motion.

If the subject flexes their hip but cannot complete full ROM, the muscle grade is considered grade 3 minus.

In very obese patients, the protruding abdomen can block the range of hip motion. In such a case, testing for grade 3 may be difficult.

In addition, some patients may be unable to lift their thigh from the seat of a chair in a sitting position, but they can flex their hip in the full range of motion in the supine position. In this case, the grade of muscle will be considered less than grade 2 plus.

6.7.4 Hip Abductor

People with severe weakness of the hip abductor must be tested in a supine position, and people with mild weakness of the hip abductor should be tested in a side-lying position.

If the hip is externally rotated, the hip flexor can substitute for hip abduction. Preventing hip external rotation is important when testing the hip abductor.

6.7.5 Knee Extensor

People with upper motor neuron lesions may lean their trunk posteriorly in order to facilitate knee extension. Detecting and preventing this compensation is important for accurate muscle test.

6.8 Assessment of Power

Adequate muscle activation speed is required for the recovery of balance (Gajdosik et al. 1999). Although a subject's power can be tested using an isokinetic dynamometer or force plate, testing using these devices is impractical in many situations.

Another method for testing the power of the lower extremities is to use mini jumping or hopping. However, in tests utilizing hopping, it may be difficult to determine whether the subject has actually hopped.

If people are unable to jump or hop, their muscle power is considered to be severely compromised. Many patients with gait disabilities also suffer from osteoporosis or musculoskeletal problems. In such cases, testing their muscle power may actually be harmful.

6.9 Summary

Muscle strength is essential to perform daily activities, and it is an important predictor of the length of a hospital stay, hospital readmission, and mortality, as well as being related to mobility and unfavorable outcomes.

The muscle strength test is used to identify weakness and detect change in muscle strength. However, it is difficult to detect changes in muscle strength without the use of a quantitative test, which also serve the purpose of increasing motivation in subjects with a gait problem.

To be used in a clinical setting, the test must be practical, which means considering the cost of the equipment, the space required for the equipment, the portability of equipment, safety (risk of injury), the duration of the measurement, and the ease of data acquisition. The manual muscle test, hand grip dynamometry, handheld dynamometry, and functional tests (e.g., the sit-to-stand test, heel raise test, etc.) are all useful in a clinical setting.

The manual muscle test is an extremely useful method for evaluating muscle strength. To be classified as grade 5, there must be a full active range of motion against gravity. After performing this full range of motion, the muscle must be able to maintain its position and resist maximal resistance. Applying maximal resistance is essential in the manual muscle test, with body weight often serving as a good means to apply maximal resistance when testing the ankle plantar flexor, for example.

Since body weight support muscles act in a closed kinetic chain throughout our daily activities, tests using a closed kinetic chain are useful for testing body weight-supporting muscles.

Postural stability is also important for testing muscle strength in people with a gait problem. One means of providing postural stability when testing body weight-supporting muscles is to have the subject rest their hands on the wall.

References

Beasley WC. Quantitative muscle testing: principles and applications to research and clinical services. Arch Phys Med Rehabil. 1961;42:398–425.

Bohannon RW. Considerations and practical options for measuring muscle strength: a narrative review. Biomed Res Int. 2019;2019:8194537.

Brown M, Avers D. Principles of manual muscle testing. In: Daniels and Worthingham's muscle testing. 10th ed. St. Louis: Elsevier; 2018a. p. 47–59.

Brown M, Avers D. Testing the muscles of the trunk and pelvic floor. In: Daniels and Worthingham's muscle testing. 10th ed. St. Louis: Elsevier; 2018b. p. 102–56.

Carr J, Shepherd R. Standing and sitting down. In: Neurological rehabilitation: optimizing motor performance. 2nd ed. St Louis: Churchill Livingstone; 2010. p. 77–94.

Davis HP, Dolny DG. A new bilateral closed chain assessment technique: methods and error analysis. Med Sci Sports Exerc. 2000;32(1):182–9.

Dvir Z. Grade 4 in manual muscle testing: the problem with submaximal strength assessment. Clin Rehabil. 1997;11:36–41.

Eliassen W, Saeterbakken AH, van den Tillaar R. Comparison of bilateral and unilateral squat exercises on barbell kinematics and muscle activation. Int J Sports Phys Ther. 2018;13(5):871–81.

Gajdosik RL, Vander Linden DW, Williams AK. Concentric isokinetic torque characteristics of the calf muscles of active women aged 20–84 years. J Orthop Sports Phys Ther. 1999;29(3):181–90.

González-Rosalén J, Benítez-Martínez JC, Medina-Mirapeix F, Pino ACD, Cervelló A, Agustín RMS. Intra- and inter-rater reliability of strength measurements using a pull hand-held dynamometer fixed to the examiner's body and comparison with push dynamometry. Diagnostics (Basel). 2021;11(7):1230.

Hébert-Losier K, Wessman C, Alricsson M, Svantesson U. Updated reliability and normative values for the standing heel-rise test in healthy adults. Physiotherapy. 2017;103(4):446–52.

Jackson SM, Cheng MS, Smith AR Jr, Kolber MJ. Intrarater reliability of hand held dynamometry in measuring lower extremity isometric strength using a portable stabilization device. Musculoskelet Sci Pract. 2017;27:137–41.

Kristensen OH, Stenager E, Dalgas U. Muscle strength and poststroke hemiplegia: a systematic review of muscle strength assessment and muscle strength impairment. Arch Phys Med Rehabil. 2017;98(2):368–80.

Lewis CL, Foch E, Luko MM, Loverro KL, Khuu A. Difference in lower extremity and trunk kinematics between single leg squat and step down tasks. PLoS One. 2015;10(5):e0126258.

Lord SR, Murray SM, Chapman K, Munro B, Tiedemann A. Sit-to-stand performance depends on sensation, speed, balance, and psychological status in addition to strength in older people. J Gerontol A Biol Sci Med Sci. 2002;57(8):M539–43.

Martin EG, Lovett RW. A method of testing muscular strength in infantile paralysis. JAMA. 1915;65(18):1512–3.

McCarthy EK, Horvat MA, Holtsberg PA, Wisenbaker JM. Repeated chair stands as a measure of lower limb strength in sexagenarian women. J Gerontol A Biol Sci Med Sci. 2004;59(11):1207–12.

Ng S. Balance ability, not muscle strength and exercise endurance, determines the performance of hemiparetic subjects on the timed-sit-to-stand test. Am J Phys Med Rehabil. 2010;89(6):497–504.

Pfister PB, de Bruin ED, Sterkele I, Maurer B, de Bie RA, Knols RH. Manual muscle testing and hand-held dynamometry in people with inflammatory myopathy: an intra- and interrater reliability and validity study. PLoS One. 2018;13(3):e0194531.

Regterschot GR, Morat T, Folkersma M, Zijlstra W. The application of strength and power related field tests in older adults: criteria, current status and a future perspective. Eur Rev Aging Phys Act. 2015;12:2.

Stark T, Walker B, Phillips JK, Fejer R, Beck R. Hand-held dynamometry correlation with the gold standard isokinetic dynamometry: a systematic review. PM R. 2011;3(5):472–9.

Thongchoomsin S, Bovonsunthonchai S, Joseph L, Chamnongkich S. Clinimetric properties of the one-leg sit-to-stand test in examining unilateral lower limb muscle strength among young adults. Int J Clin Pract. 2020;74(9):e13556.

Whitney SL, Wrisley DM, Marchetti GF, Gee MA, Redfern MS, Furman JM. Clinical measurement of sit-to-stand performance in people with balance disorders: validity of data for the five-times-sit-to-stand test. Phys Ther. 2005;85(10):1034–45.

Zawadka M, Smolka J, Skublewska-Paszkowska M, Lukasik E, Bys A, Zielinski G, Gawda P. Sex-dependent differences in single-leg squat kinematics and their relationship to squat depth in physically active individuals. Sci Rep. 2020;10(1):19601.

7 Assessment of Balance

7.1 Importance of Balance

It should be obvious that normal walking requires not only muscle strength but also the ability to balance. Severe deterioration of one's ability to balance can make walking impossible or cause falls to occur more frequently. Even if there is a slight decrease in balance ability, walking and social participation can be severely reduced, especially as it compounds with the anxiety induced by this impairment.

7.2 Role of Balance Tests

Results of balance tests may indicate the need for therapy, serve as a baseline level of function, and allow for the creation of objective documentation regarding any change in functional status (Shumway-Cook et al. 2023a). In addition, balance tests contribute to the creations of appropriate training plans while also identifying which activities are safe and unsafe.

7.3 Principle of Balance Tests

Since joints of the lower extremities continuously move during the stance period of gait (due to dynamic balance), it is necessary to employ tasks to that involve joint motion of the lower extremities when testing for balance.

So, it is possible to modify the difficulty of balance tests by altering the base of support, sensory input, speed of movement, and magnitude of movement of the center of mass.

7.4 Safety

Since there is a risk of falling and injury during balance tests, it is essential that examiners closely guard subjects in order to prevent falls. A safety belt held by another healthcare provider is the most commonly used strategy to prevent falls (Fig. 7.1).

However, safety belts do not guarantee the safety of people with a balance problem. If a healthcare provider does not adequately secure the safety belt, a fall may occur before it can be prevented. In addition, if the healthcare provider is not strong or if the subject is overweight, it may be impossible to prevent the subject from falling.

Other means, such as a wall, chair, or therapeutic mat, can also be used to increase safety. These methods are especially convenient as they are often already at hand. Also, by conducting the balance test near a wall, one direction of a potential fall can be blocked. If testing is conducted in a corner where two walls meet, two directions of a potential fall can be blocked.

If safety is uncertain even while using all the aforementioned means, the use of an overhead harness is suggested (Fig. 7.2).

Y.-S. Lee, *Task Oriented Gait Training*, https://doi.org/10.1007/978-981-97-3348-4_7

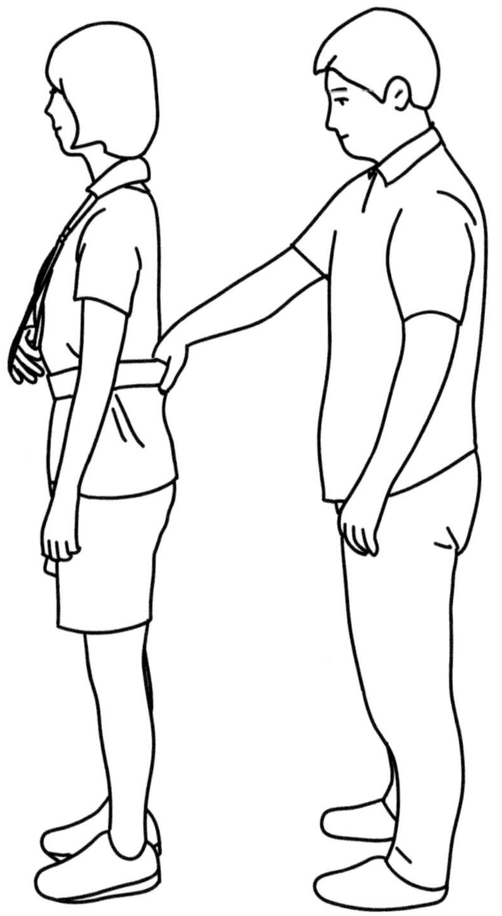

Fig. 7.1 Safety belt held by another healthcare provider

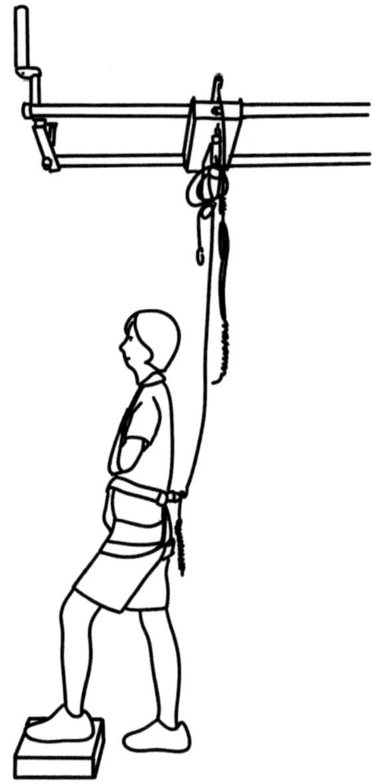

Fig. 7.2 Overhead harness

Many types of overhead harnesses are in rehabilitation. They are especially used for body weight support and fall prevention. Although an overhead harness can be useful to support a subject's body weight, it may be unnecessary if strengthening of the body weight support muscles has been completed before beginning training in a standing position. In fact, body weight support using harness system may lead to learned nonuse of the affected lower limbs. If an overhead harness is tight and is used to support the body weight of people with gait disabilities, they may become dependent on the overhead harness, which could potentially impede their movements when completing tasks.

For the sake of fall prevention, a more simple harness system can be used in place of a harness system designed for body weight support.

Although overhead harness systems are useful for preventing falls, proper use is absolutely necessary. Safety may not be guaranteed when used at home by people with cognitive dysfunction, for example.

In addition, most overhead commercial harness systems are prohibitively expensive and require an inconvenient installation process as there must be a suitable structure to which the harness system can be connected.

7.5 Subjective Perception of Balance

Perceived balance is extremely important to gait as it has a significant relationship with gait speed (Liphart et al. 2016). In addition, it strongly influences social participation (Robinson et al. 2011). People with a poor balance efficacy tend to avoid physical activity, including walking in the community (Basler et al. 2008; Bertera and Bertera 2008).

Perceived balance can be assessed via questionnaires, such as the Activities Specific

Balance Confidence (Powell and Myers 1995) or the Falls Efficacy Scale International (Tinetti et al. 1990).

However, it should be noted that there may be discrepancies between actual balance and perceived balance (Liphart et al. 2016).

If people experience anxiety due to their poor balance, they may not be able to concentrate during training tasks, so the effect of the training will be decreased.

People who underestimate their balance capacity may limit participating in challenging activities that require balance due to a fear of falling (Shumway-Cook et al. 2023b). These behaviors lead to a further decline in one's ability to balance, resulting in a vicious cycle of balance decline.

In contrast, people who overestimate their ability, such as those with anosognosia, dementia, progressive supranuclear palsy, or Huntington's disease, experience an increased fall risk (Pua et al. 2017). As such, it may be helpful to provide opportunities to do challenging tasks in a safe environment, such as with the use of an overhead harness.

7.6 Assessment of Steady-State Balance

7.6.1 Sitting Balance

A person's steady-state sitting balance can be tested while they are sitting upright. The test conditions can be changed through the use of the subject's hands or feet. If the subject cannot maintain an upright sitting position without the use of their hands, it may be useful to test whether the person can maintain an upright sitting position by propping themselves up one or both arms.

Sitting upright with one's foot in air is more difficult than placing one's feet on a wheelchair footrest or on the floor.

When testing the ability of a subject to sit upright, it is useful to measure how long they are able to maintain such a position. In addition, the alignment of the trunk is another piece of important information to take into account.

7.6.2 Standing Balance

7.6.2.1 Two-Legged Stance

Standing using both legs comfortably is the first step for testing a subject's standing balance. To conduct this test, the examiner should ask the subject to stand on both legs on a hard surface with both hands hanging comfortable at their side. Using this stance, it is possible to obtain information about whether the subject can maintain an upright standing position or not, the distance between their two feet, any asymmetry in weight distribution (alignment), and the amount of sway they demonstrate.

It may also be useful to measure the time for which they are able to maintain an upright standing position. Asymmetry in weight distribution can additionally be tested quantitatively using a standard body scale (Chap. 11).

Test can be varied using changes in sensory input and changes in the base of support. It is possible to change the sensory input by having the subject either keep their eyes open or closed, or by asking them to rotate their head. In addition, it is possible to change the characteristics of the base of support, such as by having them stand on rubber foam or on an inclined board. Moreover, feet location can be varied, such as by having the subject stand with their feet shoulder width apart, with their feet together, at a diagonal position, semi-tandem, or in a tandem position.

7.6.2.2 Clinical Tests for Sensory Interaction in Balance

For the sake of standing balance, it is important to organize and select sensory information depending on changing sensory conditions (Shumway-Cook and Horak 1986).

The Clinical Test for Sensory Interaction in Balance was developed to assess sensory organization components of standing balance. This test measures the number of seconds (with a 30-s maximum) a person can stand with both legs in six different sensory conditions that either block sensory input or provide inaccurate sensory input regarding visual and surface orientation.

Modified versions of the Clinical Test for Sensory Interaction in Balance have been developed, thus eliminating the dome condition (Allison 1995).

7.6.2.3 Single-Leg Stance Test

Since the single-leg stance test is easy to administer and does not require expensive equipment, it is useful for screening standing balance. There are many different protocols of the one-leg stance test. To improve the sensitivity of balance impairment, the test should be designed in a way that it is difficult to accomplish. Visual input must be eliminated by having the subject close their eyes. Their arms should also be folded on their chest, and having them stand on rubber foam makes the test more difficult.

In order to assess the subject's balance, not only should the time for which they can hold the stance be noted, but also any presence of sway.

7.7 Assessment of Proactive Balance

7.7.1 Sitting Balance

Sitting balance can be tested by having the subject reach out or pick up an object, such as a paper cup or wooden peg on the mat (Fig. 7.3).

Reaching can involve reaching forward, sideward, or even in a diagonal direction. Objects can be located on the mat, table, or floor. If there is any difficulty, proactive sitting balance will be impaired. Instead of using the hands, elbows can be used to touch the mat for people suffering from hemiplegia.

A modified functional reach test can be used to test the proactive sitting balance quantitatively in people with poor standing balance (Katz-Leurer et al. 2009). This test has high reliability and is responsive to improved motor performance on the paretic side (Katz-Leurer et al. 2009).

It may also be helpful to use the Motor Assessment Scale (Carr et al. 1985) or the Trunk Impairment Scale (Verheyden et al. 2004).

7.7.2 Standing Balance

7.7.2.1 Functional Reach Test

The functional reach test was developed as a quick screening for balance problems and fall risks in older adults (Duncan et al. 1990). To complete this test, subjects stand next to a wall with their feet at shoulder distance apart and one arm raised to 90° of flexion at the shoulder joint. Without moving their feet, subjects reach forward as far as possible while maintaining balance. The distance between the starting position to the final position is measured. This test has good inter-rater reliability and is predictive of falls among neurologically intact elderly subjects

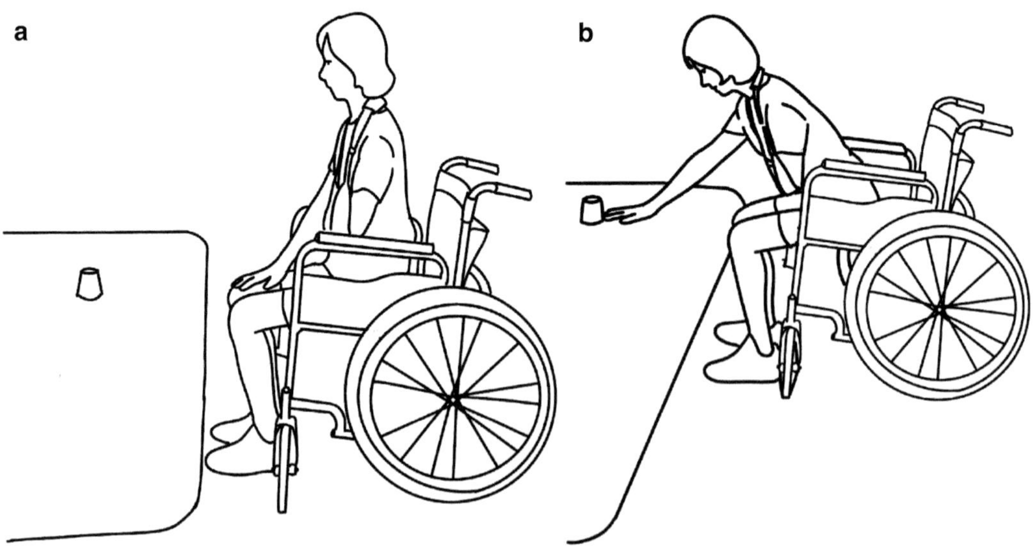

Fig. 7.3 Reaching forward to touch a paper cup on the table. The cup on the table can clarify the goal of the reaching (**a**) Starting position of reaching forward, (**b**) Final position of reaching forward

(Duncan et al. 1990). During this test, subjects must avoid rotation of the trunk. It should be noted that this test is included in the Berg Balance Scale.

In addition to having the subject reach forward, sideward and backward reaching tasks can be integrated into this test.

In this test, there is no movement of the knee joint, so it cannot be used to evaluate the ability of a subject to control their knee joint.

7.7.2.2 Step Test

The step test was developed to test dynamic standing balance after suffering a stroke (Hill et al. 1996). To administer the test, the subject should stand on the floor with both feet in front of the step. When the alarm goes off, the subject should lift one foot and place that foot on the top of the 7.5-cm-high step before then reversing the action to step back to the floor (Fig. 7.4).

Repeat this action repeatedly as quickly as possible for 15 s. Both sides must be tested, with subjects completing the test first with their non-paretic foot and then with their paretic foot. Scores for each lower limb are to be recorded separately, as well as the sum of these two scores. Test–retest reliability, validity, and responsiveness have been established (Hill et al. 1996).

The step test has many advantages in that it does not require expensive equipment and can be administered quickly and easily (Mercer et al. 2009).

However, the step test also has some limitations. Since people must stand without the assistance of walking aids and must place their foot on the top of the step, this test may be too difficult for people with a severe balance problem. In addition, its usefulness may be diminished by the floor effect.

Since the knee joint of the supporting limb maintains extension during test, it is not possible to test knee control. The result of this test may be mostly dependent on the ability of the swing limb. Also, its usefulness may be diminished by the ceiling effect.

7.7.2.3 Timed Up and Go Test

The Timed Up and Go test was developed from Up and Go test. It measures the time to stand up from a chair, walk a certain distance, turn, walk back, and sit back down in the same chair (Podsiadlo and Richardson 1991). It can be used to test dynamic balance and functional mobility.

There are many variations in the height of the chair, shape of the chair (e.g., the presence of arm rests), the distance to walk, the number of trials,

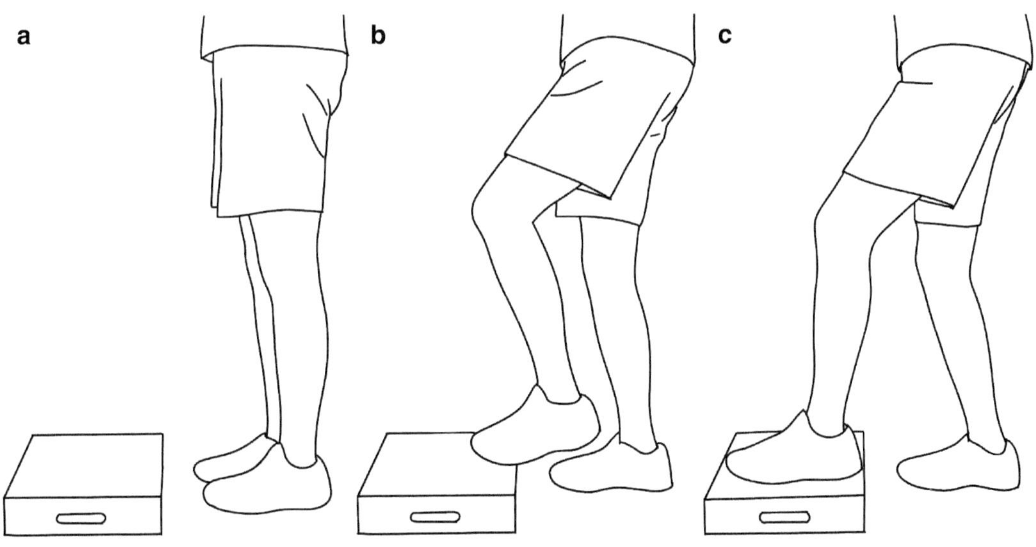

Fig. 7.4 Step test. The step test measures the number of times a foot can be placed on a 7.5-cm step and repeated for 15 seconds to return to the floor (**a**) Starting position of step test, (**b**) Midpoint of step test, (**c**) Final position of step test

dual tasks, pace (fast-paced or self-paced), and the method of turning (e.g., turning around a cone, walking to a cone, following a line on the floor, etc.).

This test is simple and does not require expensive equipment or a long time to set up. It is used to test the physical performance according to the sarcopenia criteria recommended by the European Working Group on Sarcopenia in Older People (Cruz-Jentoft et al. 2019).

7.7.2.4 Single-Leg Squat

A single-leg squat is performed by squatting from a single-leg stance and is primarily used in sports rehabilitation. Putting a stable chair behind the subject can reduce the risk of falling and injury (Fig. 7.5).

The single-leg squat is mainly used to assess movement quality, balance, stability, knee control, overall motor control, and dynamic alignment of the body (Lewis et al. 2015).

Results are evaluated by the number of repetitions completed and the degree of flexion of the lower extremity.

Most tests involving single-leg squats are visually assessed; however, it is difficult to ascertain small changes through this manner alone (Ressman et al. 2019).

Vertical ground reaction force using a force plate can provide quantitative data and increase sensitivity of the test (Eliassen et al. 2018). Since the movement of the center of mass contributes to the vertical ground reaction force of this test, vertical ground reaction force may provide useful

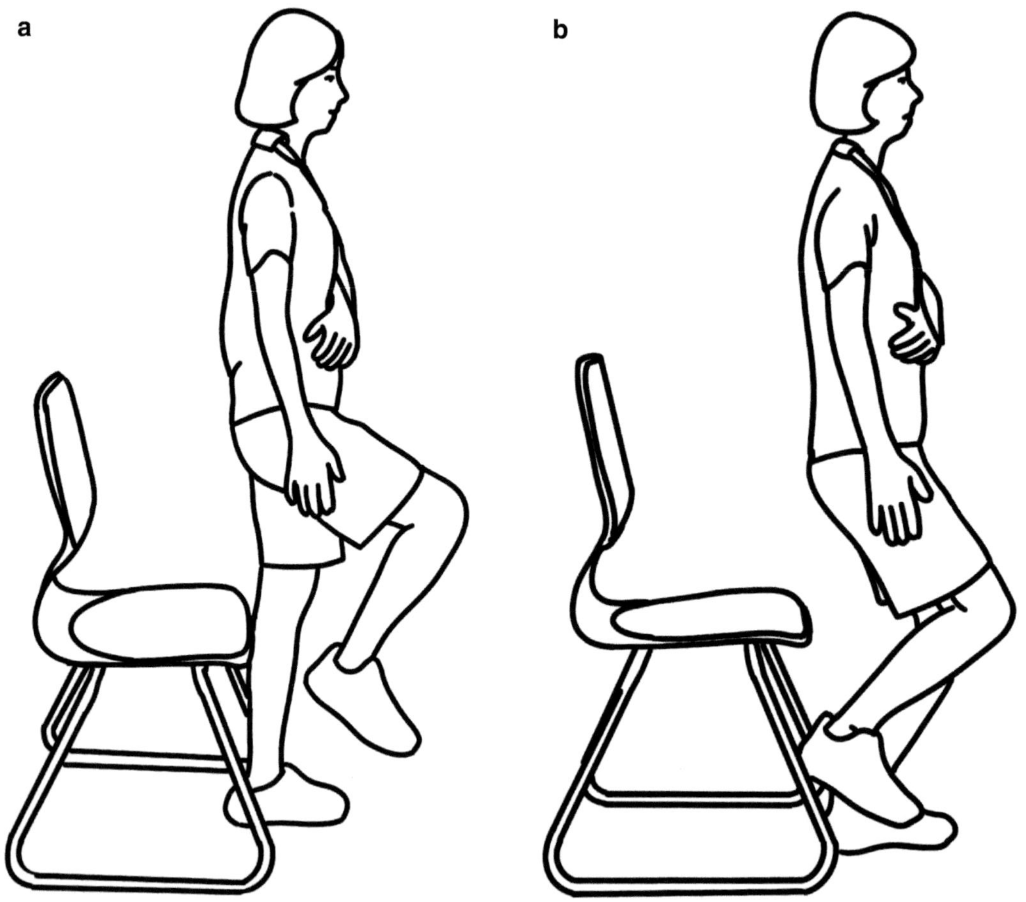

Fig. 7.5 Single-leg squat. The single-leg squat test measures the number of lower limb flexion and extension that can be repeated and degree of flexion of lower extremity while standing on one leg (**a**) Starting position of single-leg squat, (**b**) Final position of single-leg squat

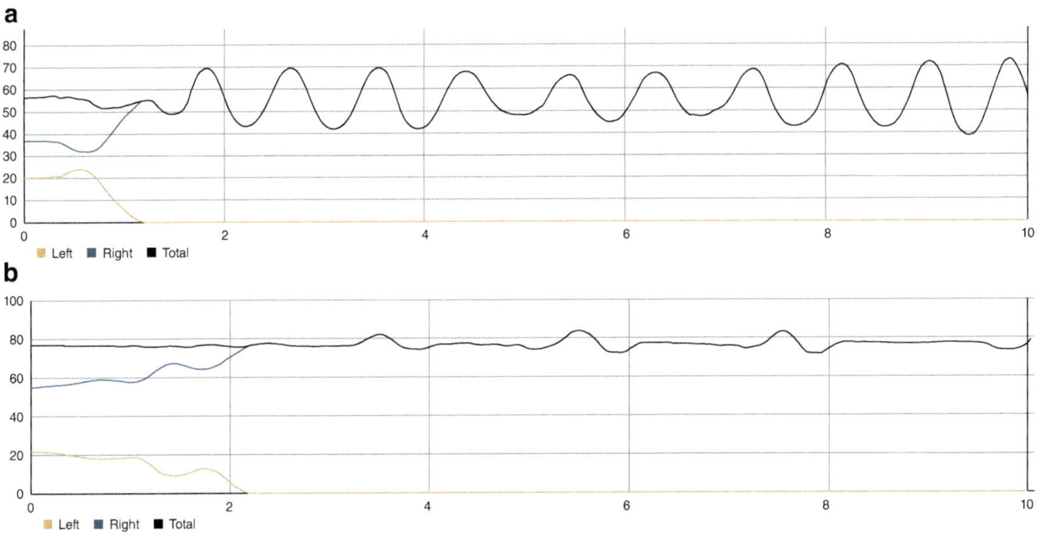

Fig. 7.6 Ground reaction force during a single-leg squat test. (**a**) Ground reaction force of a 58-year-old male subject with normal balance, (**b**) Ground reaction force of a 48-year-old female subject with hemiparesis (BBS 54)

information as to the balance ability of subjects (Fig. 7.6).

Since this test is a rather challenging task, it should only be used for people with relatively good balance.

7.8 Reactive Balance

7.8.1 Reactive Sitting Balance

A subject's reacting sitting balance can be tested using manual perturbation while they are sitting upright. It is a simple test, but the quantification of the response is difficult to ascertain.

7.8.2 Reactive Standing Balance

Reactive standing balance can be tested clinically using manual perturbation or a lean-and-release test.

The pull test is a component of the Unified Parkinson's Disease Rating Scale, scored on a 0–4 scale (Fahn et al. 1987). This test is done by pulling the shoulder of the subject from behind and grading the response.

The nudge test is a component of the Tinetti Performance-Oriented Mobility Assessment. The examiner pushes the subject's sternum lightly with the palm of their hand while the subject is standing with their feet together. Response is scored on a 0–2 scale (Tinetti 1986).

Reactive balance can also be tested by assessing the displacement of the hips (Shumway-Cook et al. 2023a). The responses are classified according to motor strategies: ankle strategy, hip strategy, and step strategy.

The lean-and-release test, which simulates a forward fall, assesses a subject's reactive stepping ability.

The examiner places their hands on the subject's shoulder, asks the subject to lean into the examiner's hands, bringing the center of mass to the limits of stability, and then unexpectedly removes their hands to cause the subject to lose their balance in a forward direction, thus eliciting a reactive step (Horak et al. 2009).

The limitation of the reactive balance test is the difficulty in controlling the perturbation force. However, this problem can be solved by using moving platforms. Although control of the perturbation force is possible with the use of a moving platform, this test is often too difficult to perform in a clinical setting, so it is only used in a research setting.

7.9 Balance Test Batteries

7.9.1 Berg Balance Scale

The Berg Balance Scale was originally used to quantitatively evaluate balance function and risk of fall in older community-dwelling adults through direct observation of their performance (Berg et al. 1989). Nowadays, the Berg Balance Scale is used for testing people suffering from a wide range of diseases, including stroke.

It is the most commonly used test in research (Lesinski et al. 2015) and in the clinical field (Korner-Bitensky et al. 2006) to evaluate balance.

The Berg Balance Scale consists of 14 items common in daily life, with each item being scored on a five-level ordinate scale ranging from 0 to 4, with 0 indicating the lowest level of function and 4 the highest level of function (Berg et al. 1989). This test has items to assess a subject's steady-state balance and proactive balance, but there is no item to test reactive balance. It needs a ruler, two standard chairs, step, and a topwatch (or wristwatch with a second hand). This test has good intra-rater reliability (Berg et al. 1989; Blum and Korner-Bitensky 2008), good internal consistency (Berg et al. 1989; Blum and Korner-Bitensky 2008), test–retest reliability (Blum and Korner-Bitensky 2008), and validity (Blum and Korner-Bitensky 2008). In addition, this test demonstrates strong correlation with the Tinetti Performance-Orientated Mobility Assessment and Timed Up and Go Test (Berg et al. 1992*).

The Berg Balance Scale has many advantages. One such advantage is the fact that this test is easy to administer and score. It also does not require expensive equipment, space, or specialized training. This test is also psychometrically sound.

Moreover, it has been found to be capable of predicting the length of stay, discharge destination, motor ability at 180 days poststroke, and disability level at 90 days post stroke (Blum and Korner-Bitensky 2008). In fact, it was reported to be the best single predictor of falls in community-dwelling older adults without neurological pathology (Shumway-Cook et al. 1997).

The limitations of the Berg Balance Scale are the floor and ceiling effects (Blum and Korner-Bitensky 2008). Due to these effects, this test may need to be conducted in conjunction with other balance measures (Blum and Korner-Bitensky 2008). Since it is insufficient on its own at assessing people with mild balance problems, it is needed to use more difficult tasks, such as hopping, to test people with a mild balance problem. In addition, as some items are subjectively evaluated by the tester, this can reduce the inter-rater reliability.

7.9.2 Balance Evaluation System Test

The Balance Evaluation System Test was developed to examine multiple aspects of balance (Horak et al. 2009). It consists of 36 items, grouped into six systems: Biomechanical Constraints, Stability Limits/Verticality, Anticipatory Postural Adjustments, Postural Responses, Sensory Orientation, and Stability in Gait. It has good reliability and correlates with other balance tests (Horak et al. 2009).

This test provides information about specific factors contributing to balance problems, and it can be used to increase the specificity of treatment (Shumway-Cook et al. 2023b).

The Mini-Balance Evaluation System Test is a shortened version of the Balance Evaluation System Test. It is composed of 14 items and can be divided into 4 subscales (anticipatory postural control, reactive postural control, sensory orientation, and gait stability). Each item is scored on a three-level ordinate scale ranging from 0 to 2 (Franchignoni et al. 2010).

Since the Balance Evaluation System Test and Mini-Balance Evaluation System Test do not have items related to sitting balance, they may be not appropriate for people with low-level functionality.

7.9.3 Community Balance and Mobility Scale

The Community Balance and Mobility Scale was developed to evaluate the balance and mobility of people with ambulatory function (Howe et al. 2006).

It is composed of 13 items, and each item is scored on six ordinate scales, with 0 indicating complete inability to perform the task and 5 indicating a most successful completion of the task.

This test requires 8-m walking track, a full flight of stairs, weights, a visual target, and a stopwatch.

As this test has more challenging tasks, it is useful for people who encounter a ceiling effect on other balance tests and can be used to detect even small balance deficits.

7.9.4 Fullerton Advanced Balance Scale

The Fullerton Advanced Balance Scale was developed for higher functioning adults to avoid the ceiling effect (Rose 2003).

It includes 10 items to test steady-state balance and proactive balance, and each item is scored on a five-level ordinate scale ranging from 0 to 4, with 0 indicating the lowest level of function and 4 the highest level of function.

Since this test has more challenging tasks, it is useful for people who encounter a ceiling effect with other balance tests.

7.9.5 Performance-Oriented Mobility Assessment

The Performance-Oriented Mobility Assessment was developed to test the gait and balance ability of elderly people (Tinetti 1986). It includes 16 items and can be divided into 2 subscales (9 balance tests and 7 gait tests). It includes items to test steady-state balance, proactive balance, reactive balance (nudge test), and sensory components. Some items are scored on a three-level ordinal scale while other items are scored on a two-level ordinal scale. This test requires a 15-foot walkway, a chair, and a stopwatch (Tinetti 1986). This test has good inter-rater reliability and is considered a good measure of fall risk in neurologically intact elderly subjects (Tinetti and Ginter 1988).

7.10 Tests Using Force Plates

Quantitative assessments are extremely important for the evaluation of people with a gait disability. One proven method of quantitatively assessing balance is through the use of a force plate. The most important parameter is related to the displacement of the center of pressure (e.g., via the area, average velocity, and amplitude). Another important parameter to take into consideration is weight distribution. Dynamic tasks can also provide kinetic information through ground reaction force.

A force plate provides real-time information on subtle changes in postural control and makes it possible to track changes in balance.

Force plates have some limitations. They are both expensive and difficult to use, so their usage is limited to research.

Although force plates are incredibly useful, it is possible to test weight distribution and ground reaction force using more simple equipment, such as a pair of body scales (Chap. 11) and a pressure sensor.

7.11 Summary

Balance tests can be conducted to evaluate steady-state balance, proactive balance, and reactive balance. To examine the many dimensions of balance, multiple tests are utilized.

Since there is always a risk of falling and injury while conducting a balance test, it is essential to prepare prevention of falls and injuries.

For the sake of testing of proactive balance, tasks that have horizontal and vertical movement of the center of mass are better than tasks that require horizontal movement only.

The Berg Balance Scale is the most commonly used test battery in both research and the clinical field to evaluate balance. This test is easy to administer and score, and it does not require expensive equipment, space, and specialized training. This test is psychometrically sound. The limitations of the Berg Balance Scale are the floor and ceiling effects.

References

Allison L. Balance disorders. In: Umphred DA, editor. Neurological rehabilitation. St. Louis: Mosby Year Book; 1995. p. 802–37.

Basler HD, Luckmann J, Wolf U, Quint S. Fear-avoidance beliefs, physical activity, and disability in elderly individuals with chronic low back pain and healthy controls. Clin J Pain. 2008;24(7):604–10.

Berg K, Sharon Wood-Dauphine S, Williams JI, Gayton D. Measuring balance in the elderly: preliminary development of an instrument. Physiother Can. 1989;41:304–11.

Berg KO, Wood-Dauphinee SL, Williams JI, Maki B. Measuring balance in the elderly: validation of an instrument. Can J Public Health. 1992;83(Suppl 2):S7–11.

Bertera EM, Bertera RL. Fear of falling and activity avoidance in a national sample of older adults in the United States. Health Soc Work. 2008;33(1):54–62.

Blum L, Korner-Bitensky N. Usefulness of the Berg balance scale in stroke rehabilitation: a systematic review. Phys Ther. 2008;88:559–66.

Carr JH, Shepherd RB, Nordholm L, Lynne D. Investigation of a new motor assessment scale for stroke patients. Phys Ther. 1985;65(2):175–80.

Cruz-Jentoft AJ, Bahat G, Bauer J, Boirie Y, Bruyère O, Cederholm T, Cooper C, Landi F, Rolland Y, Sayer AA, et al. Sarcopenia: revised European consensus on definition and diagnosis. Age Ageing. 2019;48(1):16–31.

Duncan PW, Weiner DK, Chandler J, Studenski S. Functional reach: a new clinical measure of balance. J Gerontol. 1990;45(6):M192–7.

Eliassen W, Saeterbakken AH, van den Tillaar R. Comparison of bilateral and unilateral squat exercise on barbell kinematics and muscle activation. Int J Sports Phys Ther. 2018;13(5):871–81.

Fahn S, Marsden CD, Calne DB, Goldstein M. Recent developments in Parkinson's disease, vol. 2. Florham Park: Macmillan Health Care Information; 1987. p. 153–63.

Franchignoni F, Horak F, Godi M, Nardone A, Giordano A. Using psychometric techniques to improve the balance evaluation systems test: the mini-bestest. J Rehabil Med. 2010;42(4):323–31.

Hill KD, Bernhardt J, McGann AM, et al. A new test of dynamic standing balance for stroke patients: reliability, validity and comparison with healthy elderly. Physiother Can. 1996;48:257–62.

Horak FB, Wrisley DM, Frank J. The Balance Evaluation Systems Test (BESTest) to differentiate balance deficits. Phys Ther. 2009;89(5):484–98.

Howe JA, Inness EL, Venturini A, Williams JI, Verrier MC. The Community Balance and Mobility Scale-a balance measure for individuals with traumatic brain injury. Clin Rehabil. 2006;20(10):885–95.

Katz-Leurer M, Fisher I, Neeb M, Schwartz I, Carmeli E. Reliability and validity of the modified functional reach test at the sub-acute stage post-stroke. Disabil Rehabil. 2009;31(3):243–8.

Korner-Bitensky N, Wood-Dauphinee S, Teasell R, et al. Best versus actual practices in stroke rehabilitation: results of the Canadian National Survey [abstract]. Stroke. 2006;37:631.

Lesinski M, Hortobágyi T, Muehlbauer T, Gollhofer A, Granacher U. Effects of balance training on balance performance in healthy older adults: a systematic review and meta-analysis. Sports Med. 2015;45:1721–38.

Lewis CL, Foch E, Luko MM, Loverro KL, Khuu A. Differences in lower extremity and trunk kinematics between single leg squat and step down tasks. PLoS One. 2015;10(5):e0126258.

Liphart J, Gallichio J, Tilson JK, Pei Q, Wu SS, Duncan PW. Concordance and discordance between measured and perceived balance and the effect on gait speed and falls following stroke. Clin Rehabil. 2016;30(3):294–302.

Mercer VS, Freburger JK, Chang SH, Purser JL. Step test scores are related to measures of activity and participation in the first 6 months after stroke. Phys Ther. 2009;89(10):1061–71.

Podsiadlo D, Richardson S. The timed "Up & Go": a test of basic functional mobility for frail elderly persons. J Am Geriatr Soc. 1991;39(2):142–8.

Powell LE, Myers AM. The Activities-specific Balance Confidence (ABC) Scale. J Gerontol A Biol Sci Med Sci. 1995;50A(1):M28–34.

Pua YH, Ong PH, Clark RA, Matcher DB, Lim ECW. Falls efficacy, postural balance, and risk for falls in older adults with falls-related emergency department visits: prospective cohort study. BMC Geriatr. 2017;17:291.

Ressman J, Grooten WJA, Barr ER. Visual assessment of movement quality in the single leg squat test: a review and meta-analysis of inter-rater and intra-rater reliability. BMJ Open Sport Exerc Med. 2019; 5(1):e000541.

Robinson CA, Shumway-Cook A, Matsuda PN, Ciol MA. Understanding physical factors associated with participation in community ambulation following stroke. Disabil Rehabil. 2011;33(12):1033–42.

Rose DJ. Fallproof: a comprehensive balance and mobility program. Champaign: Human Kinetics; 2003.

Shumway-Cook A, Horak FB. Assessing the influence of sensory interaction on balance: suggestion from the field. Phys Ther. 1986;66(10):1548–50.

Shumway-Cook A, Baldwin M, Polissar NL, Gruber W. Predicting the probability for falls in community-dwelling older adults. Phys Ther. 1997;77(8):812–9.

Shumway-Cook A, Woollacott MH, Rachwani J, Santamaria V. Clinical management of the patient with a postural control disorder. (Chapter11). In: Motor control: translating research into clinical practice. 6th ed. Philadelphia: Lippincott Williams & Wilkins; 2023a. p. 281–330.

Shumway-Cook A, Woollacott MH, Rachwani J, Santamaria V. Abnormal mobility. (Chapter 15). In: Motor control: translating research into clinical practice. 6th ed. Philadelphia: Lippincott Williams & Wilkins; 2023b. p. 407–39.

Tinetti ME. Performance-oriented assessment of mobility problems in elderly patients. J Am Geriatr Soc. 1986;34(2):119–26.

Tinetti ME, Ginter SF. Identifying mobility dysfunctions in elderly patients. Standard neuromuscular examination or direct assessment? JAMA. 1988;259(8):1190–3.

Tinetti ME, Richman D, Powell L. Falls efficacy as a measure of fear of falling. J Gerontol. 1990;45(6):239–P243.

Verheyden G, Mertin J, Preger R, Kiekens C, Weerdt WD. The trunk impairment scale: a new tool to measure motor impairment of the trunk after a stroke. Clin Rehabil. 2004;18:326–34.

Part III

Training

8 Principle of Gait Training

8.1 Safety

Safety is the primary concern in gait training. Holding onto a stall bar may increase the safety during gait training, but it is not a good solution as it can lead to excessive dependency on one's hands. Instead, a manual guard, wall (Carr and Shepherd 2010), chair (Carr and Shepherd 2010), mattress, corners of a wall, or an overhead harness may be better suited for the sake of increasing safety.

Guarding against falls through the use of man power could be used for safety.

To this end, a safety belt may be helpful.

However, if the subject is overweight or if the healthcare provider is not strong enough, guarding in this way is uncertain.

If used properly, an overhead harness is the most reliable safety method. In order to use an overhead harness, it must be attached to a fixed point that is higher than the subject's height.

8.2 Active Role of the Patient

It is of utmost importance that people with gait disabilities take an active role in gait training not only in a physical aspect but also in a cognitive aspect. Healthcare providers must teach sequences and the correct movements of task using verbal instructions or demonstrations.

So, people with a gait disability need time to think about whether their movement is correct or not and about any mistakes they may have made after completing the task. Then feedback from healthcare providers may be given to people with gait disability.

Using this approach, people with a gait disability can eventually complete the training independently without the need for constant supervision.

8.3 Forced Use

Although many studies showed improvement in gait after gait training, the improvements in gait were mainly accomplished by the nonaffected lower extremity. For example, many of the functional activities, such as the "stair up and down" activity or stepping over obstacles, were only possibly due to the nonparetic lower limb (Candan and Livanelioglu 2017).

However, it is important to improve paretic lower limb function, such as propulsion, to enhance gait performance in the affected lower extremity (Rowland and Lewek 2022). In addition, greater paretic limb use is related to the maintenance of improved function (Ardestani et al. 2019).

With the growing evidence of neural plasticity, treatment strategies that attempt to maximize neuroplasticity are becoming increasingly popular (Nudo 2003).

Constraint-induced movement therapy is one of the most useful strategies available to improve

Y.-S. Lee, *Task Oriented Gait Training*, https://doi.org/10.1007/978-981-97-3348-4_8

upper extremity function in people with stroke. It has shown improved arm motor function, with improvements having persisted for more than 1 year (Wolf et al. 2006). In a systematic review, there was strong evidence that constraint-induced movement therapy leads to improved quality of movement and increased use in daily life (Corbetta et al. 2015). Forced use of affected upper limbs using restraint is one of the important components of constraint-induced movement therapy as applied to the upper extremities (Morris et al. 2006; Anjos et al. 2020).

Forced use or encouragement of the avoided movements can re-engage the neglected neural circuits within the motor cortex (Kleim 2011).

The effectiveness of constraint-induced movement therapy on lower extremity motor dysfunction in people with stroke was demonstrated by a systematic review (Zhou et al. 2022).

Although constraint-induced movement therapy is extremely popular for training hemiparetic upper limbs in people with stroke, there has not been similar interest in constraint-induced movement for the lower extremities.

Forced use of the affected lower limb is important for preventing and correcting learned nonuse.

To force use of the affected lower limb, diverse methods are used, including the use of a shoe insole (Aruin et al. 2012; Candan and Livanelioglu 2017), weight on the ankle (Ribeiro et al. 2017; e Silva et al. 2017), and orthoses (Numata et al. 2008).

Shoe insoles are used to lift the unaffected lower limb and may improve weight-bearing symmetry between the two lower extremities (Aruin et al. 2012).

Some studies have reported the effectiveness of constraint-induced movement therapy on the lower extremities, but its effectiveness on gait speed and balance has been so far ambiguous in systematic reviews (Reddy et al. 2022).

In addition, constraint of the less affected lower limb during gait (whole practice) is difficult to accomplish, so there has been debate regarding the use of constraints.

Because both lower limbs are involved in gait, restraining the less impaired lower limb can interfere with normal gait pattern, so it is not recommended that the less affected lower limb be constrained (Hsu et al. 2017; Anjos et al. 2020; Abdullahi et al. 2021). Furthermore, due to the risk of falling, this method is not fully utilized in many protocols (Menezes-Oliveira et al. 2021; Anjos et al. 2020).

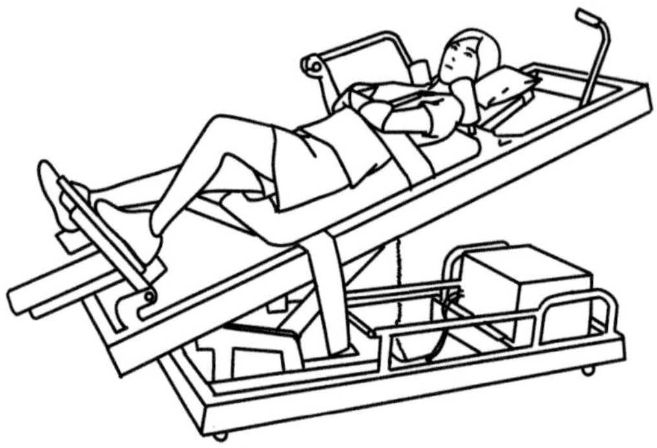

Fig. 8.1 Strengthening of the affected lower limb through the use of a sliding tilt table with placement of the unaffected lower limb on the leg raiser

Although it is difficult to perform constraint movement therapy of the lower extremities during whole practice, such as gait, it is not difficult to perform during partial practice.

Strengthening the affected lower limb through forced use can be accomplished with single-leg squats and through the use of a sliding tilt table with the unaffected lower limb on the leg raiser (Fig. 8.1).

To improve balance, training with steps (e.g., via stepping up, stepping down, stepping down and touching using the affected lower limb) can be employed.

8.4 Progressive Training

Like with other training, it is important to increase the difficulty of training to accomplish increased function in people with a gait disability. The difficulty of tasks can be changed via diverse methods, such as through the use of an inclination angle of a sliding tilt table, and by adjusting the height of steps and the distance between feet and steps. Using these methods, it is possible to minimize the risk of learned nonuse of the lower extremities.

To control the effect of gravity, many methods (such as manual support, body weight support systems, antigravity treadmills, and underwater training) are utilized. However, these methods have several limitations that can cause an overwhelming physical burden to the healthcare provider and the fact that they are inconvenient and require the use of expensive equipment.

If muscle strengthening is performed before training in standing, these methods are not necessary.

For the sake of muscle strengthening, it is important to use appropriate resistance. Since resistance is increased with the inclination angle of a sliding tilt table, changing the angle of a sliding tilt table is a thoroughly effective method of changing the resistance. Another method with which the resistance can be changed is by adjusting the degree of the flexion of joints. When training body weight support muscles, the requirement of muscle contraction increases with the degree of joint flexion.

When performing muscle strengthening exercises using a rubber band, the resistance can be changed by changing the amount that the subject stretches the rubber band.

Additionally, performing strength training in a standing position is more difficult than performing the same actions in a supine position. Changing the postural stability can be an effective method of altering the difficulty of training.

Another useful method to adjust the difficulty of training is by changing the height of the steps used. This approach requires many steps with varying heights, so it may be difficult to prepare. The training difficulty can also be increased by adjusting the distance between the foot on the floor and the foot on the top of the step.

Since the height of stairs is usually greater than that of a step, stairs can be used to perform training.

Although the difficulty of tasks can be changed according to the amount of hand use, this can lead to dependency on hand usage and learned nonuse of the affected lower limb.

For example, while training with stairs can be performed with the assistance of a subject's hands for those unable to climb stairs without this added assistance, this approach may lead to dependency on hand usage and learned nonuse of the affected lower limb (Fig. 8.2).

Hand usage can be classified as either continuous use or intermittent use. For body weight support, continuous use of the hands is employed. As such, this approach can lead to learned nonuse and musculoskeletal problems in the upper extremities. Hands can also be used for additional sensory input. Although this approach does not cause musculoskeletal problems, it must be minimized or avoided in order to regain normal gait.

Sometimes, hands can be used intermittently for safety. For example, when training by step-up, coming back to the starting position is more difficult than the initial step-up. To prevent falls, the subject may choose to use their hands during the return phase only.

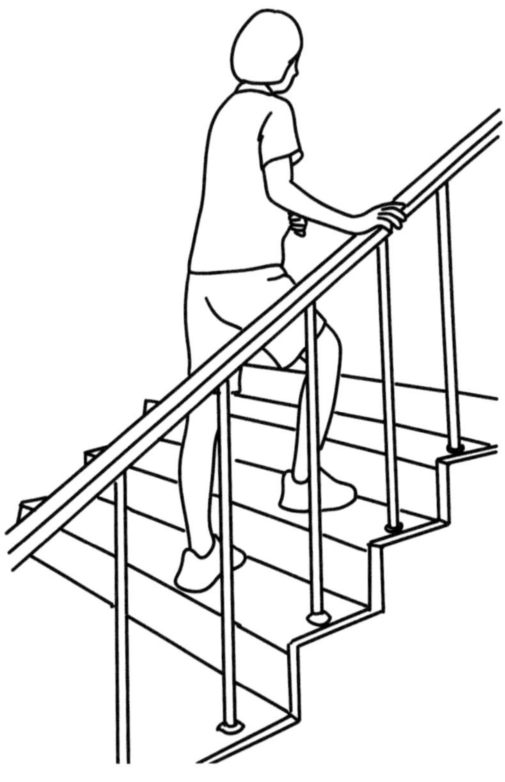

Fig. 8.2 Climbing stairs using one's hand

8.5 Feedback

In normal gait, people use their own sensory system (such as the somatosensory system or visual system) for intrinsic feedback. During gait training, extrinsic feedback may also be helpful to regain function.

External feedback to body movement can be provided by verbal cues or the guiding hands of a healthcare provider. External feedback regarding weight-bearing on the target lower extremity can be provided through the use of a bodycale or pressure sensor and display. The limitation of using a bathroom scale for extrinsic feedback is that the subject must flex their neck to observe the bathroom scale.

One downside of the continuous use of external feedback is that it can cause people to become dependent on external feedback (Shumway-Cook et al. 2023). To prevent becoming dependent on external feedback, feedback should be decreased progressively throughout the training, starting with performance feedback and decreasing the amount of performance feedback until only result feedback is provided, and then continuous feedback about results, finally reducing it to only giving summary feedback before providing no feedback at all.

8.6 Declarative Learning

Gait and relative tasks are acquired through procedural learning (nondeclarative learning), but declarative learning (instruction) may be helpful to train in these activities (such as by having the subject move their nose above their foot in a sit-to-stand task).

In a sit-to-stand task, the feet automatically move backward in healthy people. If people with a gait disability do not move their feet, it may be useful to teach this action through the use of explicit memory. Through repetitions of the task, subjects can learn to automatically move their feet during a sit-to-stand by shifting this task from explicit to implicit memory.

8.7 Specificity of Training

In order to effectively increase performance, the training should be as specific as possible (Sale and MacDougall 1981).

Training in steady-state balance does not completely transfer to dynamic balance. As such, training should also employ tasks that are related to gait.

Additionally, as body weight support muscles are activated in a closed kinetic chain during the stance period of the gait cycle, it is better to train in the closed kinetic chain tasks, such as via squats, step-ups, step-downs, and step-down touches.

8.8 Intensity

Intensity is a cornerstone for the promotion of neuroplastic changes and long-lasting functional improvement.

The intensity of training can be expressed by the number of repetitions, the total treatment time, and the level of difficulty (Dobkine 2008).

8.8.1 Amount of Training

It is well known that the training dosage is closely related to the result of training or, in other words, the level of daily activity of people with a stroke (Kwakkel et al. 2004), the balance of elderly people (Lesinski et al. 2015), and the strength of the elderly (Borde et al. 2015).

Training dosage can be expressed by the repetition number (such as the number of step-ups or steps) or by the total training time.

Although high-intensity training and practicing stepping are the most important factors of mobility outcomes and stepping activity (Hornby et al. 2020), the daily dosage of lower extremity exercises post stroke in comprehensive stroke units is fewer than 300 repetitions (Scrivener et al. 2012).

Increasing the amount of training with one-to-one training is impractical due to cost. Other methods, such as supervised group training that includes circuit training and independent training (with or without equipment), are required. Studies have also shown that it is beneficial to add small amounts of supervised sessions to mainly unsupervised intervention (Lacroix et al. 2017).

Training without supervision, such as via home-based exercise programs, could reduce the costs of training. Additionally, training at home is likely to facilitate participation (Lacroix et al. 2017).

8.8.2 Difficulty of Tasks

The difficulty of tasks can be assessed using performance and subjective analysis. In step-up training, the performance of the step-up action, such as its smoothness or the movement of the center of mass, can be used to determine its difficulty. However, such parameters require special equipment. So, taking into account the success rate of tasks may be a more practical route. To prevent people with a gait disability from experiencing excessive frustration, a more than 80% success rate may be a good target to reach because if a subject feels that a specific task is too difficult, their motivation may decrease.

In aerobic training, Borg's scale is used to assess the subjective difficulty of a task, and a score of 12–14 of 20 (somewhat difficult) is usually the target intensity. In gait training, subjective analysis can be used to select a task that is appropriately somewhat difficult for the subject.

8.9 Motivation

Many people with a gait disability have little motivation and a poor threshold for frustration. However, the experience of success can improve a patient's motivation. By setting a target time of 5 seconds, subjects who can maintain a standing position for only 7 seconds can experience the feeling of success. Additionally, this may be helpful by providing information about the positive aspects of their health status (such as a subject's relatively good muscle strength) in people with a gait disability.

If people perceive an improvement in their impairment or function, their motivation may increase. With this in mind, using objective and quantitative assessments that can measure small changes in impairment and function can be helpful.

In addition, it is helpful to explain the reason behind specific tasks designed to regain gait. If people accept the importance of training in a specific task, their motivation for that training can increase.

8.10 Variable Training

Variable training is important as it allows trained tasks to be used in the real world. It is possible to make variations in the training by changing the distance between the subject's feet, the location of their feet (e.g., parallel, diagonal, semi-tandem, and tandem), the speed of task performance, and virtual targets (such as in a computer game).

8.11 Detraining

The effects of training fade away with time (Toulotte et al. 2006). To maintain an adequate training effect, continuous monitoring and exercise is required. Since gait training is a lifelong process, easy and cost-effective strategies are needed.

8.12 Gait Training Cycles

Training can be divided into three stages: the initial stage, the refinement stage, and the maintenance stage (Fig. 8.3).

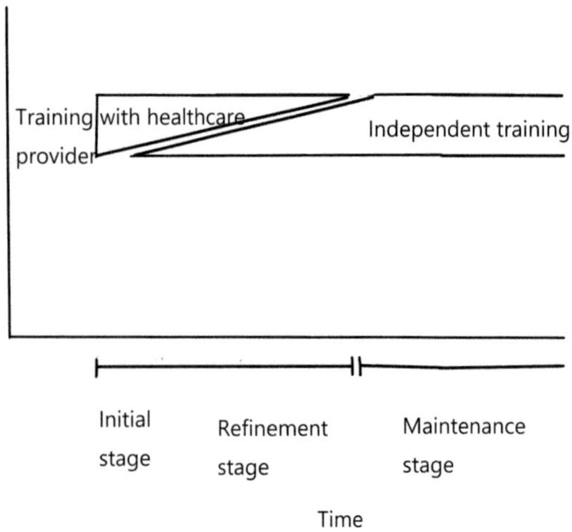

Fig. 8.3 Stages of training

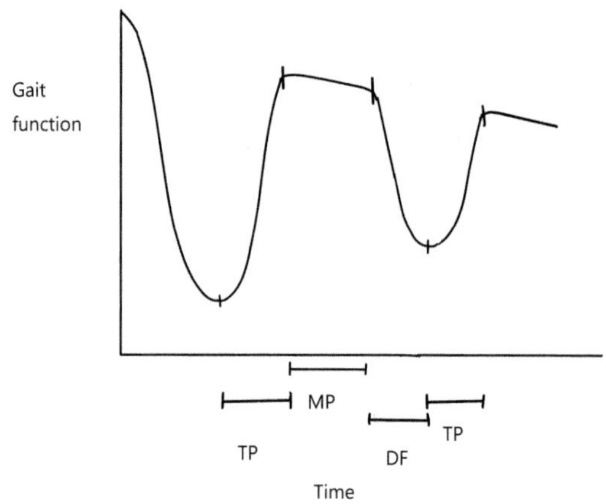

Fig. 8.4 Cycles of gait training. *TP* training period, *MP* maintenance period, *DF* deterioration of gait function

In the initial stage of training, people cannot perform tasks correctly, their performance is generally abnormal, and there is a higher risk of falls and injuries. During this stage, healthcare providers must train the subjects to perform the tasks and correct any abnormal performance that they observe. However, some tasks can be conducted independently by the subject, such as strengthening of the hip internal rotator. Through training progression, tasks can be made more difficult over time.

In the refinement stage, subjects tend to have more knowledge about the tasks and are able to correct their own abnormalities during training. Tasks can also be altered for more effective training, such as through changes in the base of support (e.g., soft or slippery ground), changes of sensory input (e.g., having the subject keep their eyes closed), and by performing dual tasks. Training can be done in a group setting or in an unsupervised setting. In this stage, there is an increase in the performance of tasks.

During the maintenance stage, there is no improvement in performance or even a slight decrease in performance. This is the stage at which subjects need to perform tasks that have been mastered in the previous stage in order to maintain their acquired function.

If function has been found to have decreased significantly, it may be necessary for the subject to resume the gait training cycle again (Fig. 8.4).

8.13 Facilitate Engagement with the Exercise Program

Exercising continuously to maintain health and gait function is difficult. To solve this problem, several strategies may be helpful in facilitating engagement in the exercise program: feedback on performance, gamification of exercise, and an exercise log. However, in many cases, the effects of these strategies have been found to be unsatisfactory.

Community programs may be helpful in facilitating engagement with the exercise program. Many characteristics of community programs, such as the encouraging atmosphere, social interaction, and games in groups, may be helpful. Community programs may also facilitate the social participation of people with a gait disability. This aspect of training will be mentioned in more detail in a following chapter.

8.14 Summary

It is obvious that training strategies must be consistent with current knowledge. However, there are some gaps between the current knowledge and clinical practice. Thus, it is essential that current knowledge be incorporated into the training plan. The best gait training should not only be effective, it should be safe, cost-effective, and easily performed.

Restraint of the unaffected upper limb is one of the most important components of constraint-induced movement therapy for the upper extremities. Although restraining the less affected lower limb is difficult to accomplish, constraint movement therapy of the lower extremities during whole practice, such as in gait training, is not so difficult to perform during partial practice.

During gait training, extrinsic feedback may be helpful for regaining function. However, continuous use of external feedback can cause subjects to become dependent on external feedback. To prevent this, feedback should be decreased alongside the progression of training.

Since training effects are determined by the amount of training, it is important to increase the amount of training. Unsupervised, independent training may be a useful strategy toward increasing the amount of training.

References

Abdullahi A, Truijen S, Umar NA, Useh U, Egwuonwu VA, Van Criekinge T, Saeys W. Effects of lower limb constraint induced movement therapy in people with stroke: a systematic review and meta-analysis. Front Neurol. 2021;12:638904.

Anjos SD, Morris D, Taub E. Constraint-induced movement therapy for lower extremity function: describing the LE-CIMT protocol. Phys Ther. 2020;100(4):698–707.

Ardestani MM, Henderson CE, Hornby TG. Improved walking function in laboratory does not guarantee increased community walking in stroke survivors: potential role of gait biomechanics. J Biomech. 2019;91:151–9.

Aruin AS, Rao N, Sharma A, Chaudhuri G. Compelled body weight shift approach in rehabilitation of individuals with chronic stroke. Top Stroke Rehabil. 2012;19:556–63.

Borde R, Hortobágyi T, Granacher U. Dose-response relationships of resistance training in healthy old adults: a systematic review and meta-analysis. Sports Med. 2015;45(12):1693–720.

Candan SA, Livanelioglu A. Effects of modified constraint-induced movement therapy for lower limb on motor function in stroke patients: a randomized controlled study. Int J Theor Phys. 2017;4:269–77.

Carr J, Shepherd R. Training motor control, increasing strength and fitness and promoting skill acquisition (Ch 2). In: Neurological rehabilitation: optimizing motor performance. 2nd ed. St. Louis: Churchill Livingstone; 2010. p. 15–55.

Corbetta D, Sirtori V, Castellini G, Moja L, Gatti R. Constraint-induced movement therapy for upper extremities in people with stroke. Cochrane Database Syst Rev. 2015;10:CD004433.

Dobkine BH. Training and exercise to drive poststroke recovery. Nat Clin Pract Neurol. 2008;4(2):76–85.

e Silva EMGS, Ribeiro TS, da Silva TCC, Costa MFP, da Costa Cavalcanti FA, Lindquist ARR. Effects of constraint-induced movement therapy for lower limbs on measurements of functional mobility and postural balance in subjects with stroke: a randomized controlled trial. Top Stroke Rehabil. 2017;24:555–61.

Hornby TG, Henderson CE, Holleran CL, Lovell L, Roth EJ, Jang JH. Stepwise regression and latent profile analyses of locomotor outcomes poststroke. Stroke. 2020;51(10):3074–82.

Hsu CJ, Kim J, Roth EJ, Rymer WZ, Wu M. Forced use of the paretic leg induced by a constraint force applied to the nonparetic leg in individuals post-stroke during walking. Neurorehabil Neural Repair. 2017;31(12):1042–52.

Kleim JA. Neural plasticity and neurorehabilitation: teaching the new brain old tricks. J Commun Disord. 2011;44(5):521–8.

Kwakkel G, van Peppen R, Wagenaar RC, Dauphinee SW, Richards C, Ashburn A, Miller K, Lincoln N, Partridge C, Wellwood I, Langhorne P. Effects of augmented exercise therapy time after stroke: a meta-analysis. Stroke. 2004;35(11):2529–39.

Lacroix A, Hortobágyi T, Beurskens R, Granacher U. Effects of supervised vs. unsupervised training programs on balance and muscle strength in older adults: a systematic review and meta-analysis. Sports Med. 2017;47(11):2341–61.

Lesinski M, Hortobágyi T, Muehlbauer T, Gollhofer A, Granacher U. Effects of balance training on balance performance in healthy older adults: a systematic review and meta-analysis. Sports Med. 2015;45(12):1721–38.

Menezes-Oliveira E, Matuti GDS, de Oliveira CB, de Freitas SF, Kawamura CM, Lopes JAF, Arida RM. Effects of lower extremity constraint-induced movement therapy on gait and balance of chronic hemiparetic patients after stroke: description of a study protocol for a randomized controlled clinical trial. Trials. 2021;22:463.

Morris DM, Taub E, Mark VW. Constraint-induced movement therapy: characterizing the intervention protocol. Eura Medicophys. 2006;42(3):257–68.

Nudo RJ. Adaptive plasticity in motor cortex: implications for rehabilitation after brain injury. J Rehabil Med. 2003;41:7–10.

Numata K, Murayama T, Takasugi J, Oga M. Effect of modified constraint-induced movement therapy on lower extremity hemiplegia due to a higher-motor area lesion. Brain Inj. 2008;22(11):898–904.

Reddy RS, Gular K, Dixit S, Kandakurti PK, Tedla JS, Gautam AP, Sangadala DR. Impact of constraint-induced movement therapy (CIMT) on functional ambulation in stroke patients—a systematic review and meta-analysis. Int J Environ Res Public Health. 2022;19(19):12809.

Ribeiro TS, Chaves da Silva TC, Carlos R, de Souza e Silva EMG, Lacerda MO, Spaniol AP, Lindquist ARR. Is there influence of the load addition during treadmill training on cardiovascular parameters and gait performance in patients with stroke? A randomized clinical trial. NeuroRehabilitation. 2017;40:345–54.

Rowland DM, Lewek MD. Linking gait mechanics with perceived quality of life and participation after stroke. PLoS One. 2022;17(9):e0274511.

Sale D, MacDougall D. Specificity in strength training: a review for the coach and athlete. Can J Appl Sport Sci. 1981;6(2):87–92.

Scrivener K, Sherrington C, Schurr K. Exercise dose and mobility outcome in a comprehensive stroke unit: description and prediction from a prospective cohort study. J Rehabil Med. 2012;44(10):824–9.

Shumway-Cook A, Woollacott MH, Rachwani J, Santamaria V. Motor learning and recovery of function (Chapter 2). In: Motor control: translating research into clinical practice. 6th ed. Philadelphia: Lippincott Williams & Wilkins; 2023. p. 22–45.

Toulotte C, Thevenon A, Fabre C. Effects of training and detraining on the static and dynamic balance in elderly fallers and non-fallers: a pilot study. Disabil Rehabil. 2006;28(2):125–33.

Wolf SL, Winstein CJ, Miller JP, Taub E, Uswatte G, Morris D, Giuliani C, Light KE, Nichols-Larsen D, EXCITE Investigators. Effect of constraint-induced movement therapy on upper extremity function 3–9 months after stroke: the EXCITE randomized clinical trial. JAMA. 2006;296(17):2095–104.

Zhou M, Tu Y, Cui J, Gao P, Yi T, Wang J, Hao Q, Li H, Zhu T. Effect of constraint-induced movement therapy on lower extremity motor dysfunction in post-stroke patients: a systematic review and meta-analysis. Front Neurol. 2022;13:1028206.

9 Muscle Strengthening

9.1 Relationship Between Strength and Gait

Although some studies have reported that strengthening exercises did not lead to changes in gait (Judge et al. 1993; Ouellette et al. 2004), there is also robust evidence that strengthening exercises improve gait. These discrepancies can be explained by the nonlinear relationship between muscle strength and walking speed (Buchner et al. 1996).

Since gait does not require strong muscle contractions of the lower extremities, strengthening does not necessarily lead to an improvement in gait in people with mild muscle weakness. However, it can improve gait in people with severe or moderate muscle weakness.

9.2 Mechanisms of Muscle Strengthening

9.2.1 Lower Motor Neuron Lesions

The regaining of strength in patients with lower motor neuron lesions is achieved through progressive resistance training. In cases of lower motor neuron lesions, an increase in strength is attained through alterations in the firing characteristics of anterior horn cells and muscle hypertrophy.

9.2.2 Upper Motor Neuron Lesions

The recovery of strength in patients with upper motor neuron lesions is achieved through the workings of several mechanisms, including diaschisis, disinhibition, and plastic changes in synapses. Among these mechanisms, changes in synapses are the most important for regaining muscle strength as induced by training. However, achieving changes in synapses requires numerous repetitions.

9.3 Principles of Muscle Strengthening

9.3.1 Appropriate Amount of Resistance

Strengthening is typically accomplished through progressive resistance strength training. To ensure effective training, it is crucial to determine and apply the appropriate amount of resistance.

9.3.1.1 Lower Motor Neuron Lesions

In cases of lower motor neuron lesions, the amount of resistance can be determined by either the percentage of a subject's one-repetition maximum or the repetition number. The percentage of a one-repetition maximum with free weights is commonly used for strengthening (Ada et al.

Y.-S. Lee, *Task Oriented Gait Training*, https://doi.org/10.1007/978-981-97-3348-4_9

2006; Duncan et al. 2003; Ouellette et al. 2004). To use this method, information about the one-repetition maximum is required. Determining a subject's one-repetition maximum necessitates multiple trials of muscle contraction with different weights, which can be time-consuming and somewhat inconvenient. For high-intensity strengthening programs, people can use 70–79% of their one-repetition maximum, perform 7–9 repetitions per set, complete 2–3 sets per exercise, and engage in 2 sessions per week (Borde et al. 2015). Since there is no need for multiple trials of muscle contraction, determining the appropriate resistance using the repetition number is more convenient than relying on the percentage of a one-repetition maximum. When using the repetition number to determine the appropriate resistance, it is necessary to adjust the resistance to the next level when the repetition number falls outside the target range during training. In healthy individuals, a repetition number of 10–15 is frequently used. The target number is determined by the individual's health status, with 10–20 repetitions generally being utilized by people with gait disabilities. If the repetition number exceeds 20, the amount of resistance must be increased, and if the repetition number falls below 10, the amount of resistance should be decreased. This method is very convenient and time-saving.

9.3.1.2 Upper Motor Neuron Lesions

Individuals with upper motor neuron lesions find it challenging to perform selective contractions, adjust the intensity of muscle contractions, and coordinate muscle contractions effectively. Because of this difficulty, descending signals may overflow to other muscles, resulting in incorrect movements. Thus, it is crucial to minimize or avoid these overflows. Excessive resistance can also lead to an overflow of descending signals, making it essential to adjust resistance levels to prevent this issue. In individuals with severe paresis, controlled eccentric muscle contractions can be more challenging than concentric contractions, and there may be a fear of sudden collapse while standing. Performing strengthening exercises in a lying-down position can reduce anxiety and help people with a gait disability to focus on the muscle contractions themselves. Therefore, when selecting training methods for muscle strength, it is imperative to ensure that these methods do not lead to incorrect movements, such as unnecessary associated movements or uncontrolled contractions.

9.3.2 Postural Stability

In a stable position, individuals can generate more peak force (van den Tillaar and Larsen 2020). Therefore, exercises performed in a lying-down position are beneficial for strength training, especially for people with balance problems or upper motor neuron lesions. When conducting strengthening exercises in a sitting or standing position, using a wall for hand support can enhance postural stability and exercise efficiency.

9.3.3 Training Specificity

The body weight support muscles of the lower extremities are typically engaged in closed kinetic chains of muscle contractions during the stance period of the gait cycle. Training in a closed kinetic chain, such as by using one's body weight, can be a more effective training method than training in an open kinetic chain, such as by using free weights.

9.3.4 Control of the Effect of Gravity

Although gravity remains constant, its effects can be altered by changing the posture or alignment of one's body segments. Gravity-minimized postures are used to train grade 2 muscles. In many muscles of the extremities, side-lying postures serve as gravity-minimized positions. However, for some muscles, such as axial muscles, hip internal rotators, and hip external rotators, an upright posture is the gravity-minimized position. An upright posture is particularly effective for training these muscles.

9.3.5 Mode of Strength Training

Various methods are employed for muscle strengthening, including functional electrical stimulation, free weights, elastic bands, body weight exercises, and the use of a sliding tilt table. For individuals with mild-to-moderate muscle weakness, body weight exercises are a very convenient option for strength training. However, in cases of subjects with severe weakness (less than grade 3 on the manual muscle test), special equipment like a sliding tilt table can be helpful for strength training.

9.4 Facilitation of Muscle Contraction

When there is no voluntary motion of body segments (manual muscle strength grades 0 and 1), it is necessary to facilitate muscle contraction. Several methods can be employed for this purpose, including sensory stimulation, functional electrical stimulation, changes in joint position, weight-bearing, bilateral simultaneous muscle contraction, and the passive motion of joints.

9.4.1 Functional Electrical Stimulation

Functional electrical stimulation (FES) is a commonly used strategy for muscle strengthening in individuals with upper motor neuron lesions (UMNL) (Kesar et al. 2009; Awad et al. 2015; Yang et al. 2018).

9.4.2 Weight-Bearing

Weight-bearing stimulates Golgi's tendon organs, skin somatosensory receptors, and muscle spindles. Consequently, it promotes the contraction of body weight support muscles (Duysens et al. 2000). In individuals with severe motor impairment, weight-bearing on the affected lower limb while standing can be very challenging. However, it can be easily achieved using a tilt table or a sliding tilt table.

9.4.3 Change of Joint Alignment

In people with upper motor neuron lesions, it is possible to promote or suppress muscle contraction by changing the alignment of the joints. The extension of the hip joint promotes the contraction of the knee extensor muscle, and the flexion of the hip joint inhibits the contraction of the knee extensor muscle (Lewek et al. 2006).

9.5 Strengthening with a Closed Kinetic Chain Exercise

Exercise via a closed kinetic chain in standing position is widely used in sports rehabilitation and gait training. It offers several advantages for strengthening body weight support muscles, including the ability to strengthen multiple muscles simultaneously, train multi-joint coordination, and is more functional because body weight support muscles work in a closed kinetic chain during gait. In addition, this type of exercise does not require equipment. However, it may be too challenging for people with severe weakness.

9.5.1 Bridging

9.5.1.1 Bridging with Two Legs

Bridging is done in a supine position. Initially, the subject must flex the hip joints and knee joints while maintaining a neutral position of the hip joint in the transverse plane. Subjects then place their feet on the floor.

Using a ball between the knees may help maintain a neutral position of the hip joint in the transverse plane. It is better to train hip control in the transverse plane to perform bridging without holding anything between the knees.

The subject then raises their hips off the floor as high as possible and maintains that position for several seconds. Finally, they return to the starting position and repeat this exercise (Fig. 9.1).

This exercise can strengthen the back extensors, hip extensors, and hamstrings. Some individuals, especially those with hemiparesis, may perform bridging with external rotation of the

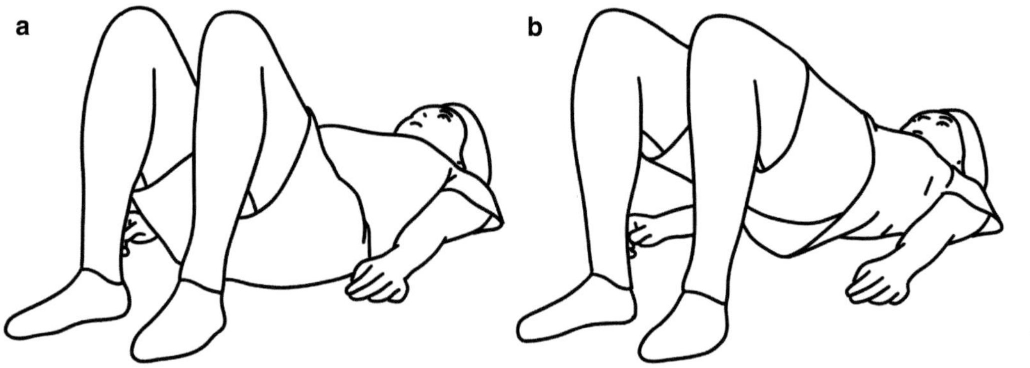

Fig. 9.1 Bridging with two legs: (**a**) starting position of bridging with two legs; (**b**) final position of bridging with two legs

affected lower limb. This should be corrected as continuing training in this manner may lead to learned nonuse and thus negatively impact recovery. Correcting this can involve teaching the correct exercise method, reducing the degree of muscle contraction, and strengthening the hip internal rotators of the affected lower limb.

Bridging offers several advantages, such as not requiring a transfer to another space, not posing a risk of falling, and presenting the opportunity to experience weight-bearing on the sole of the foot in a supine position. It may be too difficult for individuals with severe weakness of lower extremity muscles or hip joint flexion contracture. This problem can be alleviated using a pressure sensor system under the sole of the foot and display. Since muscle contraction during bridging is expressed as a change in ground reaction force, this can provide external feedback to people with gait disabilities.

9.5.1.2 Bridging with One Leg

Bridging with one leg requires not only stronger muscle contraction of the back extensors, hip extensors, and hamstrings, but also hip internal rotators.

Start by flexing the hip and knee joint of the affected limb and placing affected foot on the floor. Then flex the contralateral hip joint while maintaining the knee joint extension. Finally, lift hip as high as possible (Fig. 9.2).

In some individuals, this exercise may be too challenging. In such cases, modifying the exercise can make it possible for individuals with moderate weakness. Initially, lift the buttocks with both legs, and then lift one leg and maintain that position. By increasing the time spent maintaining that position, it is possible to strengthen the aforementioned muscles.

9.5.2 Sit-to-Stand

The sit-to-stand is crucial for mobility and requires stronger muscle contractions than overground walking. In a sit-to-stand exercise, the vertical movement of the body is achieved by the hip and knee extensors. Therefore, it is a valuable exercise for strengthening the body weight support muscles of the lower limbs.

In a sit-to-stand exercise, quantifying the resistance and the amount of exercise is straightforward. The amount of resistance is determined by the height of the seat, making it easy to adjust during sit-to-stand exercises (Rodosky et al. 1989). The amount of exercise can be expressed using the repetition number of sit-to-stand movements.

For people with balance problems, performing sit-to-stand without using their hands may be too challenging or their performance may deteriorate. By resting their hands on the wall, people can do a sit-to-stand safely, and this also allows individuals with gait disabilities to focus more on the sit-to-stand movement (Fig. 9.3).

Therefore, people with gait disabilities can contract their muscles more effectively. While safety bars, therapeutic tables, or chair armrests

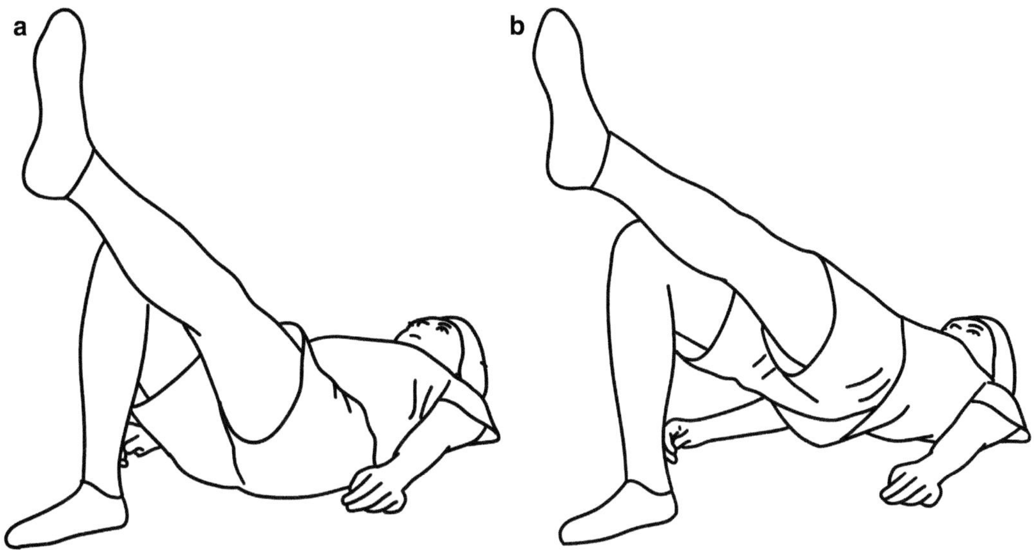

Fig. 9.2 Bridging with one leg: (a) starting position of bridging with one leg; (b) final position of bridging with one leg

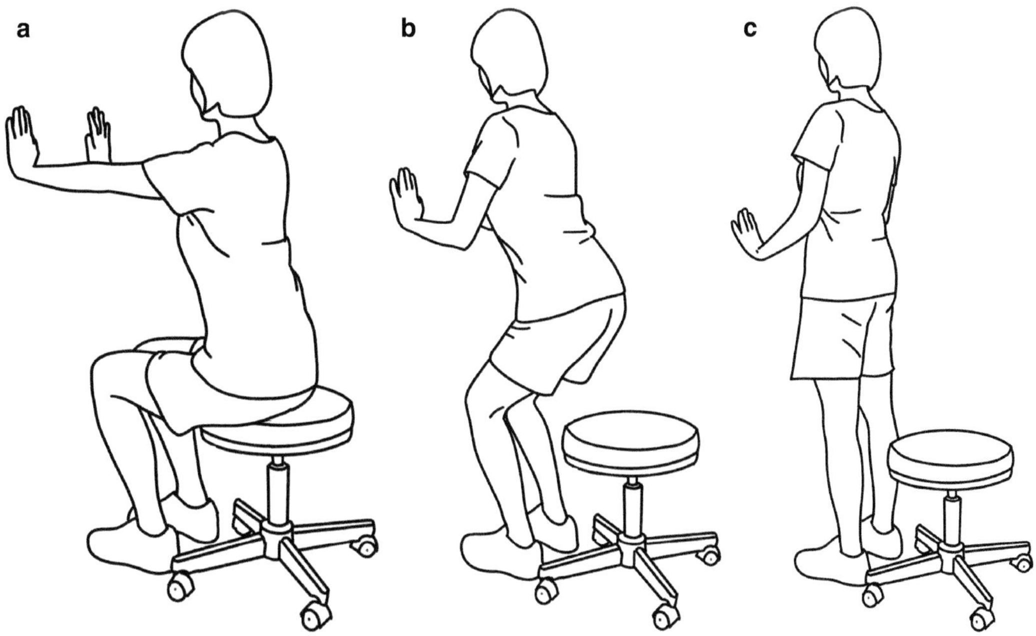

Fig. 9.3 Sit-to-stand exercise with two legs. By touching the wall with hands, it is possible to do sit-to-stand safely. (a) Starting position, (b) Midpoint of sit-to-stand, (c) Final position

can enhance safety, they may lead individuals to rely on their upper extremities for body weight support, reducing the effectiveness of the sit-to-stand exercise and potentially causing musculoskeletal problems in the upper limbs.

The difficulty of sit-to-stand is determined not only by the muscle strength of the body weight support muscles but also by the height of the chair seat, the subject's balance, and the speed of the sit-to-stand motion.

The height of the chair seat is an important determinant of the difficulty of the sit-to-stand exercise. As the height of the chair seat increases, the required muscle contraction decreases, and the number of repetitions can increase. Conversely, with a decrease in the height of the chair seat, the required muscle contraction increases, and the number of repetitions decreases. Therefore, it is necessary to adjust the height of the chair seat to enable people with gait disabilities to repeat the sit-to-stand exercise to the target number, which is between 10 and 20.

For individuals with insufficient muscle strength (i.e., those able to achieve only a repetition number less than 10), a chair with a higher seat, which reduces the requirement of muscle contraction needed to lift the body, may be helpful for performing sit-to-stand movements. As strength improves, the seat height can be lowered. One simple method for increasing the seat's height is by placing a flat object on the top of the seat.

If individuals can perform the sit-to-stand exercise more times than the target number, it is necessary to decrease the height of the chair. It is possible to increase resistance by shifting body weight to the targeted lower limb (Fig. 9.4).

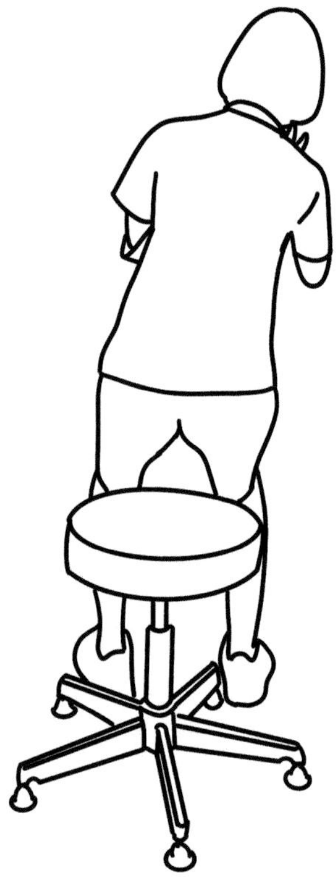

Fig. 9.4 Sit-to-stand exercise with weight shifted to the right lower limb

Providing feedback to individuals with gait disabilities regarding the degree of weight shift is possible using a standard body scale or a pressure sensor.

The requirement for lower extremity force during a rapid sit-to-stand movement can be reduced by generating and transferring momentum between the upper body and the total body (momentum strategy). Therefore, rapid sit-to-stand motions may reduce the effectiveness of the exercise and increase the risk of musculoskeletal problems, such as back pain. Hence, a slow and controlled sit-to-stand motion (force control strategy) is beneficial for strengthening the body weight support muscles of the lower extremities. In the force control strategy, the center of mass has to move toward the feet. Instructing individuals to move their "nose over the toe" may be helpful in achieving this (Shumway-Cook et al. 2023).

The sit-to-stand exercise offers numerous advantages. First, it does not require special devices and can be performed anywhere using a chair. It also does not demand much preparation time, is a functional task frequently performed in daily life, and is safe because the chair prevents individuals from collapsing to the floor. If the subject rests their hands on the wall, the exercise becomes even safer.

However, there are some limitations to the sit-to-stand exercise. If there is asymmetric impairment between the two lower limbs, especially in people with upper motor neuron lesions, individuals may use the less affected lower limb more, potentially leading to learned nonuse of the affected lower limb. Many individuals with hemiparesis exhibit low activation of the tibialis anterior (TA) on the affected side, and compensatory excessive activation of the TA and quadriceps muscles in the unaffected limb (Cheng et al. 2004). Additionally, excessive hip flexion during sit-to-stand movements may inhibit knee extension, especially in individuals with upper motor neuron lesions.

It may be helpful to force the use of the affected lower limb by placing the foot of the unaffected lower limb on the top of a step, positioning the unaffected foot anterior to the affected foot. Visual feedback concerning the amount of weight-bearing on the unaffected foot may also be beneficial.

9.5.3 Squat with Two Legs

Squat exercises can be used to strengthen the antigravity muscles in the lower extremities. Squatting is a very useful method for strengthening the lower extremity body weight support muscles in healthy individuals. It is widely used in sports rehabilitation and in the community for ordinary people. The standard squat is initiated from a standing position by flexing the joints of both lower limbs to the target point.

However, there is a risk of knee injury when performing squats using incorrect methods. Therefore, it is important to avoid anterior movement of the knee joint to prevent knee injuries. Despite efforts to prevent knee injuries, some people may experience knee problems after performing squat exercises. As a result, squats may not be suitable for individuals with gait disabilities.

The risk of knee injury can be reduced by modifying the exercise method. Squats with a chair are safer than conventional squats (Flanagan et al. 2003). They eliminate the risk of falling and help individuals perform the exercise using the correct technique. Chair squats are especially useful for people with gait disabilities because they are safer than conventional squats (Fig. 9.5).

Squats with a chair offer another benefit. The chair's seat can serve as the target for the squat exercise. People can clearly determine when they have reached the target point by touching the chair's seat with their buttocks. This exercise resembles sit-to-stand exercises. If the buttocks only touch the chair, it is considered a squat with a chair. If the buttocks momentarily rest on the chair, it becomes a sit-to-stand exercise.

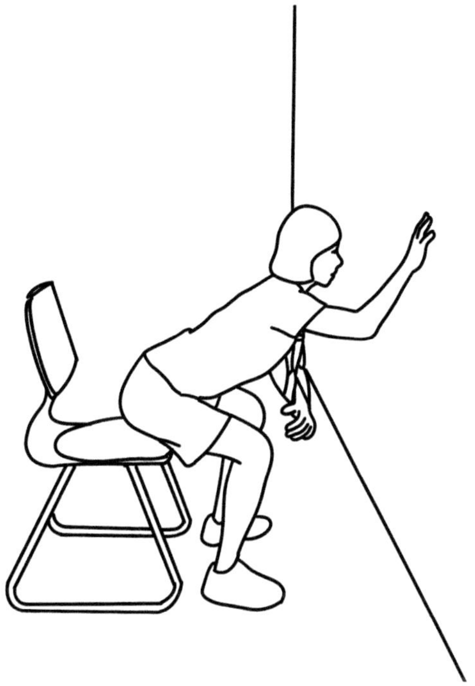

Fig. 9.5 Chair squats with both limbs

Another modification involves using the hands for stability. Postural stability can be achieved by touching the wall with hands during squats, making the squat easier to perform (Fig. 9.6).

If the number of repetitions is less than the target number, it is possible to increase the height of the target by placing a flat object on the top of the seat. Conversely, if the number of repetitions exceeds the target number, it is necessary to lower the height of the seat or place a step under the feet. Squat exercises do not require special equipment and can be performed without much preparation time. However, in individuals with asymmetric lower limb problems, squats may lead to learned nonuse of the more affected lower limb. To prevent learned nonuse, it may be helpful to place the less affected foot on a step, putting the less affected lower extremity at a mechanical disadvantage. Another method is to place the less affected limb on a body weight scale. By using a body scale, people with a gait disability can receive feedback regarding the degree of body

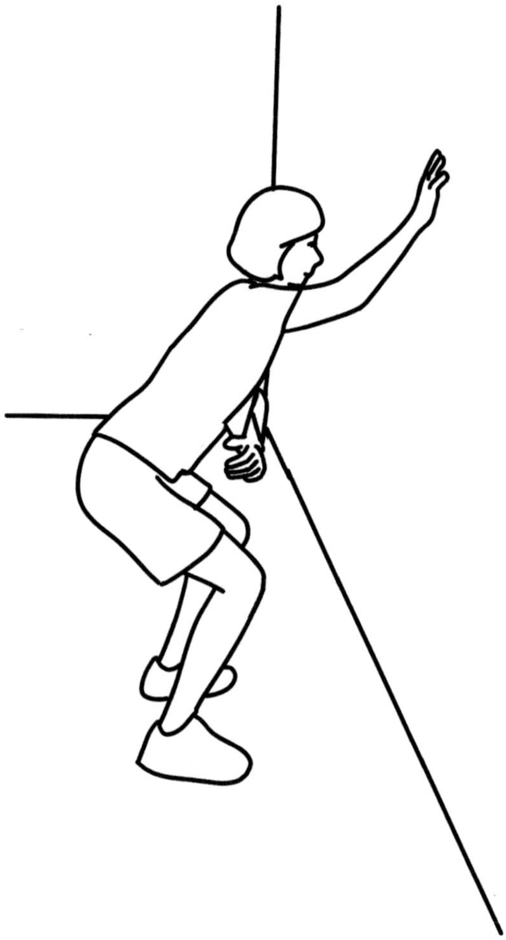

Fig. 9.6 Squat exercise with wall touch using two legs

weight support for the less affected lower limb. People should aim to gradually decrease the body weight support of the less affected lower extremity.

9.5.4 Single-Leg (Mini) Squat

Eccentric contraction is more challenging than concentric contraction, especially for people with upper motor neuron lesions. Eccentric contraction can be trained using squat exercises. Squat exercises that involve both lower extremities in people with asymmetric impairments may lead to learned nonuse, and forced use may be necessary to prevent this. Training with one leg is more effective, but in cases of danger, training with both lower extremities is preferable.

The single-leg mini squat can be used to strengthen body weight support muscles in the lower limb and may be a useful training method for preventing learned nonuse in individuals with asymmetric impairments (Fig. 9.7).

This exercise is referred to by many different names, including the unilateral squat, and it has primarily been used in sports training (Speirs et al. 2016).

Postural stability can be increased by touching the wall with a hand during the single-leg squat. After regaining knee control using the single-leg squat, training can progress to the single-leg squat without hand support. It is necessary to minimize hand usage to transition to the single-leg squat without hand support. If people rely on leaning against a wall during the single-leg squat, it may become a habit and hinder progress to the next step of training (Fig. 9.8).

To minimize hand usage, it is essential to train with more weight-bearing on the heel. Shifting weight to the heel promotes a more vertical posture and reduces hand usage (Fig. 9.9).

Although the single-leg mini squat is extremely useful for people with asymmetric impairments, it can be challenging to assess the amount of flexion in the lower extremity (e.g., in the hip, knee, and ankle joints). Since ground reaction force changes with the flexion and extension of the lower limb, it is possible to provide feedback regarding the flexion of the lower extremity using ground reaction force (Fig. 9.10).

9.5.5 Heel Lift

Heel lift is a very useful exercise for increasing the strength of the ankle plantar flexors, and it is widely used in clinical practice. Heel lifts can be performed with one leg or both legs, depending on the strength of the ankle plantar flexors.

People with moderate-to-severe exercise capacity can perform heel lifts with both legs. To begin, stand with both lower limbs, feet comfortably apart in front of a wall while facing it. Lift the arms and rest the hands on the wall. Then lift both heels simultaneously as high as possible and return to the starting position. Repeat these movements as many times as possible.

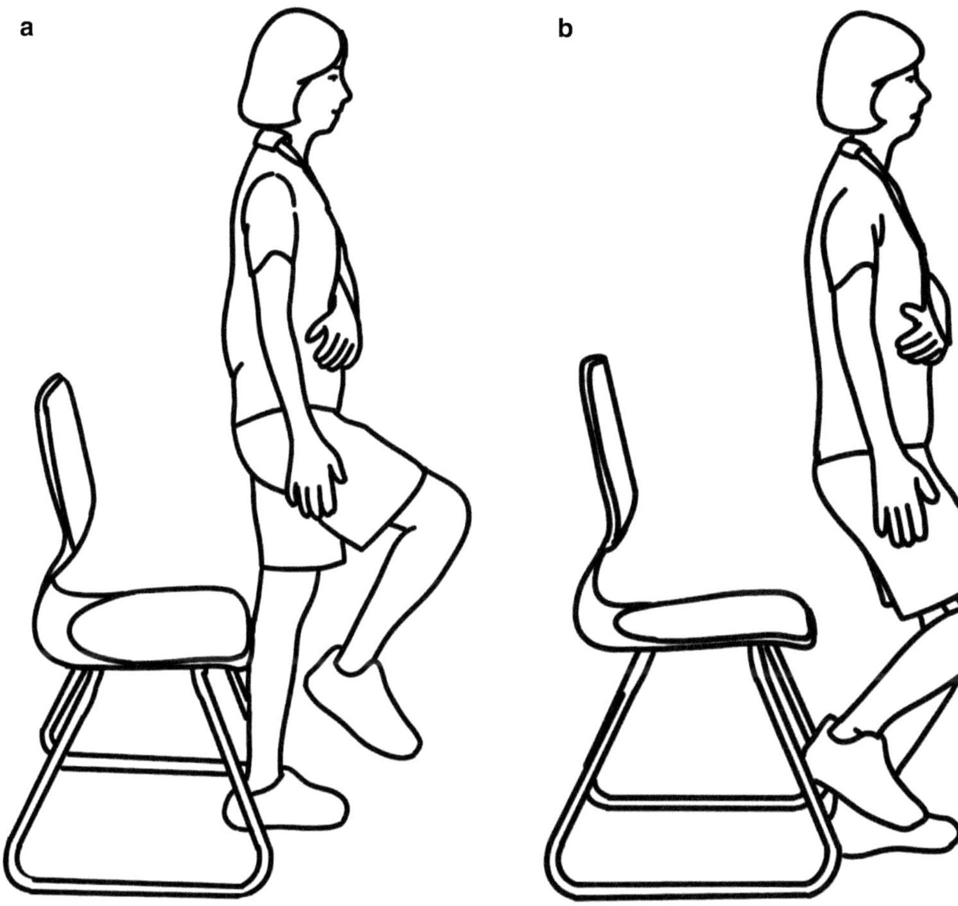

Fig. 9.7 Single-leg squat: (**a**) lower limb extension; (**b**) lower limb flexion

If individuals cannot fully lift their heels or cannot continuously repeat the exercise 20 times, continue exercising in the same method. If individuals can fully lift their heels more than 20 times using both legs, they can progress to heel lifts using both legs with weight shifting. If they have symmetric weakness, they can alternate weight shifting to both sides. If they have asymmetric weakness, they can shift their weight more to the affected side (Fig. 9.11).

When performing heel lifts, it is essential to move through a sufficient range of motion. If individuals lift their heels within a minimal range of motion due to weakness, that signals that the resistance is too great to perform the exercise correctly.

In people with lower motor neuron lesions, it is very useful to strengthen the ankle plantar flexors by doing heel lifts using both legs with a weight shift to the affected side. However, in people with upper motor neuron lesions, this may be an ineffective method for strengthening the ankle plantar flexors of the affected leg. In such cases, it may be helpful to place the unaffected foot on the seat of a chair and anterior to the affected foot (Fig. 9.12).

Since the unaffected foot is at a mechanical disadvantage in this position, it makes weight shifting to the affected side easier. To prevent the trunk from moving forward, rest the fingers on the wall with elbow extension and shoulder flexion at 90°. Mechanical disadvantage increases the higher the position of the foot, the further forward the foot is placed, and the more vertical the person's posture becomes.

Some people may not be able to increase muscle strength with heel lifts in a standing position.

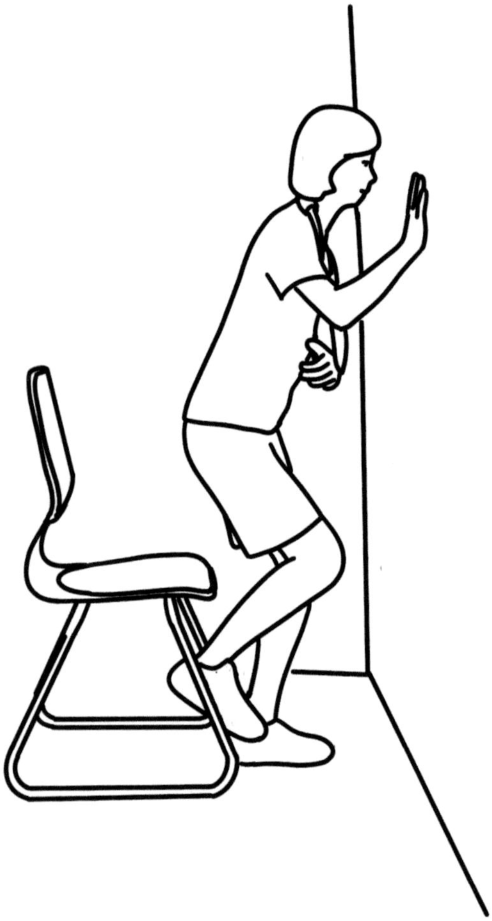

Fig. 9.8 Leaning against a wall during the single-leg squat

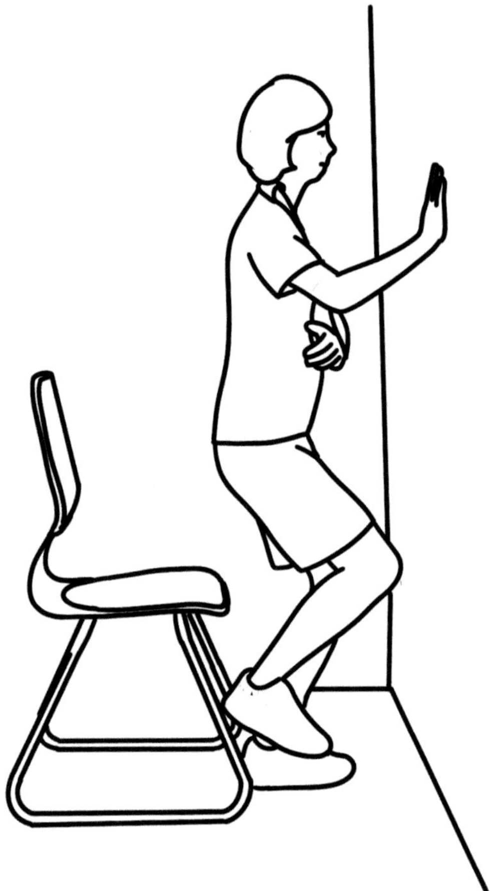

Fig. 9.9 Single-leg squat with vertical posture

In such cases, it may be helpful to train with an elastic band or a sliding tilt table.

If the muscle strength of individuals is grade 3 minus or stronger, heel lifts can be done with one leg, which is more effective than heel lifts using two legs. In order to perform one-leg heel lifts, start by standing with feet comfortably apart in front of a wall while facing the wall. Lift your arm and rest your hand on the wall. Then lift one leg and maintain that position. Lift the heel of the weight-bearing leg as high as possible (Fig. 9.13). Return to the starting position and repeat these movements as many times as possible.

People with poor standing balance may tilt to the lateral side and fall down while performing heel lifts with one leg. In such cases, it is helpful to do heel lifts at the corner of a wall (Fig. 9.14).

This alleviates the fear of falling and prevents actual tilting and falling.

It is important to ensure that the resistance is appropriate. Although people may be able to perform heel lifts with one leg, if the range of ankle motion is very limited due to muscle weakness, modification of training is required.

Heel lifts have many advantages as they do not require special equipment or much time to prepare for the exercise. However, people with poor standing balance or severe muscle weakness may find it impossible to perform heel lifts.

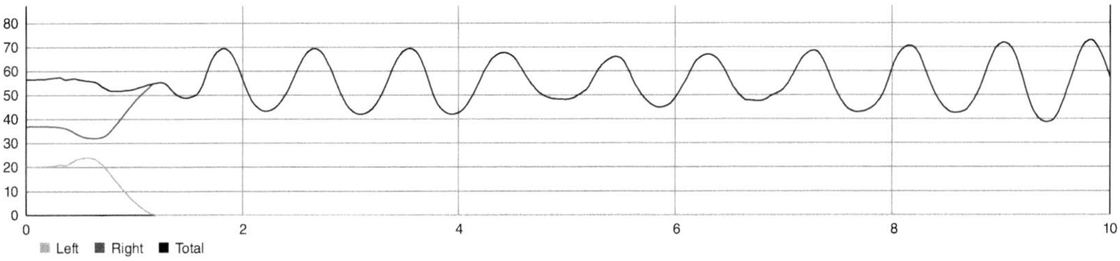

Fig. 9.10 Change of ground reaction force during single-leg squats

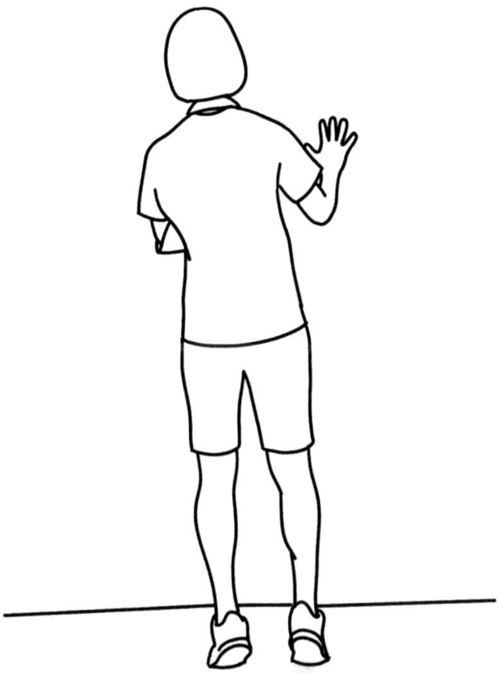

Fig. 9.11 Heel lift with weight shift using two legs

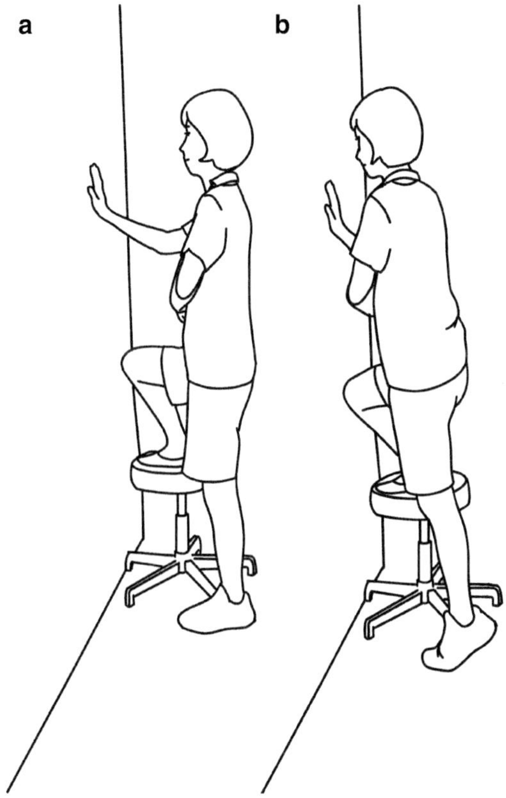

Fig. 9.12 Heel lift using two legs with mechanical disadvantage of unaffected leg. The use of the normal leg can be made more difficult by placing the foot of the normal leg high: (**a**) starting position; (**b**) final position

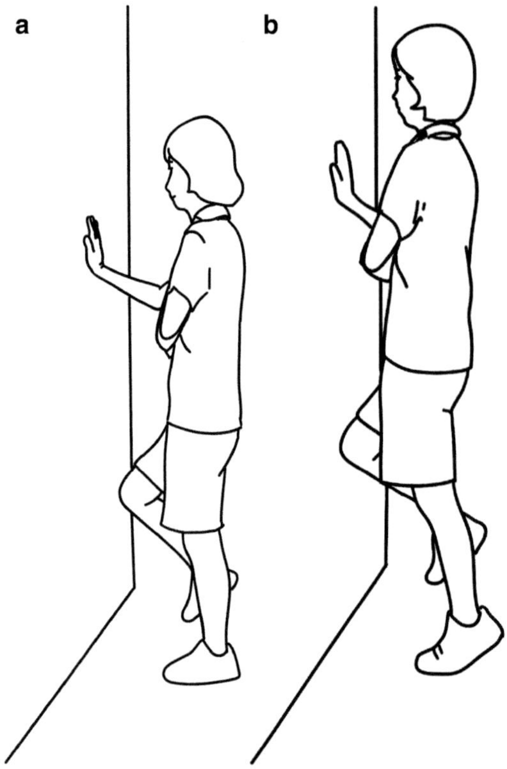

Fig. 9.13 Heel lift using one leg: (**a**) starting position; (**b**) final position

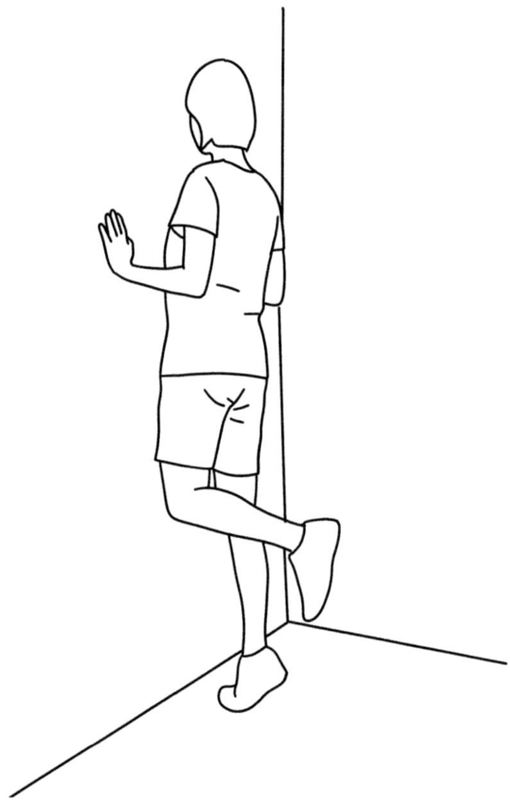

Fig. 9.14 Heel lift at the corner of a wall using one leg

9.6 Exercise with Elastic Band

Exercise with an elastic band offers many advantages. First of all, elastic bands are not expensive, and they do not require much space for storage or time to prepare for the exercise. They are portable and can be used anywhere, including in bed, making them especially useful for people with mobility problems. Additionally, they can be used on nearly all muscles in the body, and exercise using an elastic band is considered relatively safe.

However, its biomechanics differ from exercises utilizing gravity. The relationship between joint angle and resistance varies from exercises with body weight in a standing position (such as in sit-to-stand movement or squats). Gravity remains constant, whereas the resistance of an elastic band changes according to the degree of stretching. When exercising body weight support muscles with one's body weight in a standing position (similar to the action of body weight support muscles during gait), the requirement for muscle contraction decreases as the muscle shortens because the center of mass is closer to the joint axis as the muscle shortens. In contrast, the requirement for muscle contraction increases with muscle shortening when using an elastic band because the resistance of the rubber band increases as the length of the rubber band also increases (Fig. 9.15).

Since the amount of resistance is based on the subjective feeling of the user, it can be difficult to determine the exact degree of resistance. This challenge can be more pronounced in people with poor motivation or cognitive dysfunction.

Quantifying resistance can be a challenging task but not an impossible one. For example, it can be supplemented by using a traction dynamometer. Combining an elastic band with a trac-

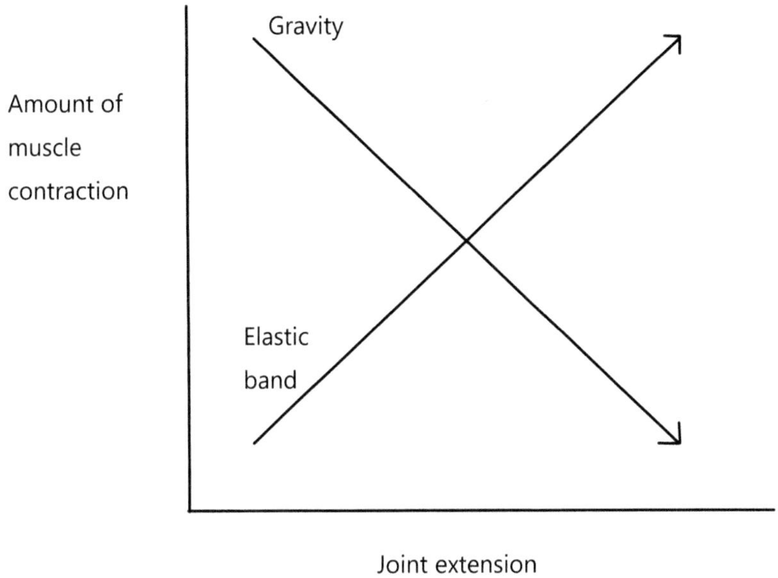

Fig. 9.15 Relationship between joint extension and muscle contraction

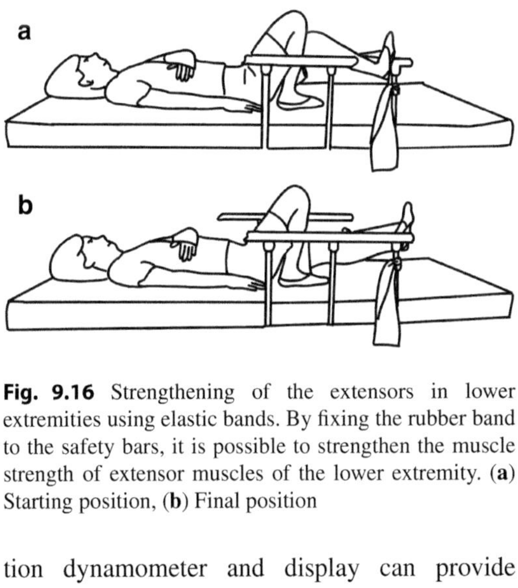

Fig. 9.16 Strengthening of the extensors in lower extremities using elastic bands. By fixing the rubber band to the safety bars, it is possible to strengthen the muscle strength of extensor muscles of the lower extremity. (**a**) Starting position, (**b**) Final position

tion dynamometer and display can provide real-time information about resistance. Nowadays, there are commercial products available that provide feedback through visual displays.

It is possible to strengthen not only individual muscles but also multiple antigravity muscles simultaneously using total (hip and knee joint) flexion and extension of the lower limbs in a supine position (Fig. 9.16).

Exercises using a rubber band for each muscle will be described in the section covering the strengthening of individual muscles.

9.7 Exercise with a Sliding Tilt Table

9.7.1 Components of the Sliding Tilt Table

The sliding tilt table consists of a supporting frame, tilting frame, sliding top, a motor to adjust the inclination angle of the tilting frame, a friction-reducing mechanism designed to minimize friction between the tilting frame and the sliding top, a leg raiser, a goniometer, a device for adjusting the range of motion, and footplates that can be rotated upward or downward (Fig. 9.17). The sliding tilt table was used for the first time in patients with severe burns (Trees et al. 2003). The sliding tilt table can be used not only for patients with severe burns, but also for those with severe muscle weakness or paralysis.

9.7.2 Characteristics of a Sliding Tilt Table

A sliding tilt table combines the benefits of a conventional tilt table, commonly used for individuals who cannot stand independently, with those of a leg press machine often found in fitness clubs. It offers a low-friction environment for iso-

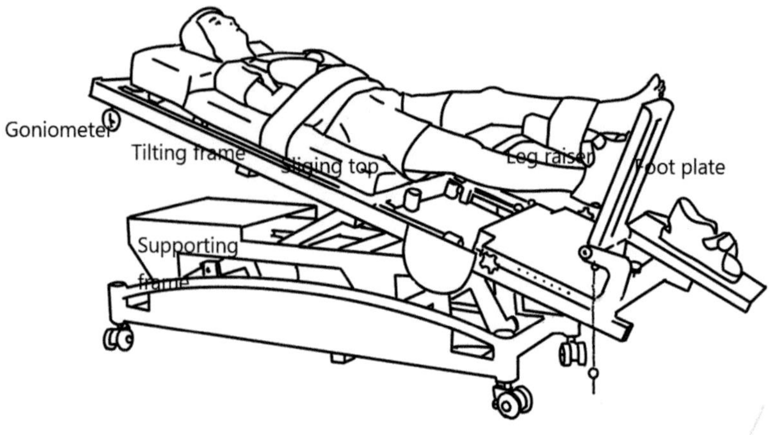

Fig. 9.17 Sliding tilt table

tonic exercises while maintaining postural stability in a lying-down position. This combination makes it a valuable tool in both rehabilitation and strengthening programs for people with severe impairments.

9.7.3 Advantages of a Sliding Tilt Table

Exercise with a sliding tilt table has several characteristics that make it highly effective for strengthening the body weight support muscles of the lower limbs, especially the hip extensors and knee extensors. This type of exercise is particularly beneficial for individuals with severe lower limb weakness, those who are overweight, and with individuals with balance problem, cognitive impairments, or low motivation.

The advantages of the sliding tilt table are as follows:

Ease of Use for Severely Weak Individuals: The sliding tilt table allows people with severe weakness to perform exercises with minimal muscle contraction. The body and sliding top can be moved with just one finger to be at a lower inclination angle, making it accessible even to those with very severe weakness.

Stability for Balance Problems: People with balance problems can benefit from the sliding tilt table as it provides a stable and secure posture. The exercises are performed in a lying-down position, reducing the risk of falls or instability.

Cognitive-Friendly: The flexion and extension of the lower extremities on a sliding tilt table involve familiar movements, making it suitable for individuals with cognitive impairments. The simplicity of the exercise helps participants focus on the task at hand.

Motivation and Progress Tracking: Individuals with low motivation can find success and see clear progression with the sliding tilt table. Changes in the inclination angle and the number of repetitions offer tangible markers of improvement.

Safety: Exercising on a sliding tilt table is inherently safe. The Velcro straps secure the individual in a lying-down position, reducing the fear of falling during training. Moreover, eccentric muscle contractions can be trained safely on a sliding tilt table.

Functional Training: The sliding tilt table allows for functional training because it mimics the flexion and extension of the lower extremities while they are bearing weight, mimicking the movements that occur frequently in daily life.

Multi-Muscle Engagement: It enables the simultaneous strengthening of multiple muscles, providing a comprehensive workout.

Forced Use of Affected Limbs: The addition of a leg raiser on a sliding tilt table allows for the forced use of the affected lower limb, which can be crucial for rehabilitation.

9.7.4 Setup of a Sliding Tilt Table Before Exercise

Before transferring an individual to a sliding tilt table, it is necessary to ensure that the tilting frame is parallel to the ground to facilitate a safe and easy transfer. After transferring an individual to the sliding tilt table, it is important to position them on the sliding top with their back lying down, and secure their body with Velcro straps to prevent falls. Maintaining heel contact with the footplate is essential throughout body weight support muscle strengthening, with the exception of heel lifts. In the case of training with a single lower limb, the unaffected (or less affected) lower limb must be placed on the leg raiser to enforce the use of the affected lower limb (Fig. 9.18).

Using leg support is crucial to promote the forced use of the affected lower leg.

9.7.5 Training with One Lower Leg

To strengthen the antigravity muscles of the lower limb, the total flexion and extension of the limb (i.e., the hip and knee flexion, and ankle joint) are crucial. Training with both lower limbs is suitable for individuals with symmetric weakness, while training with a single lower limb is appropriate for those with asymmetric weakness. Some healthcare providers train people with asymmetric impairment in lower limbs using both lower limbs when training with the sliding tilt table. This training can lead to learned nonuse

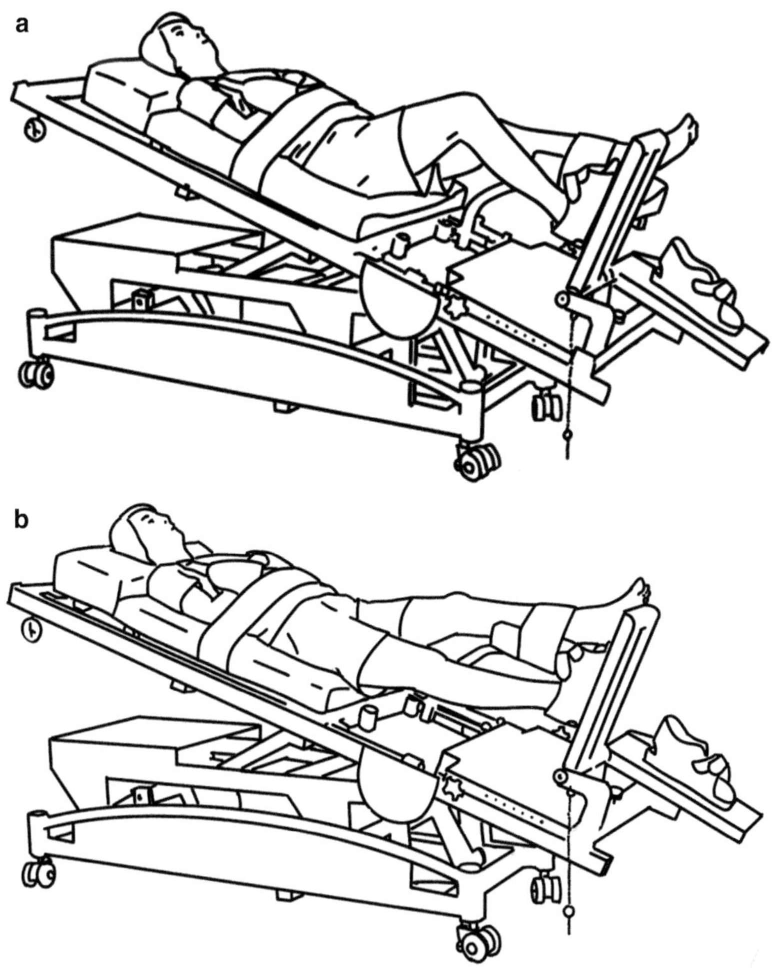

Fig. 9.18 Forced use of an affected lower limb with leg raiser while training with sliding tilt table. By placing the normal lower extremity on the leg raiser, it is possible to prevent the normal lower extremity from participating in pushing up the trunk. (**a**) Starting position, (**b**) Final position

of the more affected lower limb. Thus, it is recommended to train using the hemiparetic lower limb only, even if people have similar weakness in both lower limbs.

9.7.5.1 Training with Correct Motion

Similar to other exercises, it is essential to perform exercises with controlled (slow) and correct movements. If there is incorrect movement during the exercises, it is important to stop the incorrect movement and correct it. Education, plus adjusting the settings of the sliding rehabilitation machine, including the inclination angle, can help correct improper movements.

It is important to ensure that individuals understand the correct movement of the task and the importance of performing exercises correctly. Incorrect exercise techniques can become habits and lead to abnormal gait patterns.

If a task is too challenging for individuals, people may perform it incorrectly or use compensatory strategies. It is crucial to appropriately adjust the task's difficulty to be appropriate for each individual. The task's difficulty can be adjusted by modifying the range of motion or inclination angle. Decreasing the range of motion (i.e., reducing the maximum angle of flexion) can make it easier to extend from a flexed position, and reducing the inclination angle can also facilitate extension from a flexed position.

9.7.5.2 Amount of Resistance

The amount of resistance should be individualized based on the individual's disease, the severity of impairment, and their overall health condition. Strengthening exercises for individuals with upper motor neuron lesions may require a higher number of repetitions. There is no specific recommendation for the amount of resistance based on clinical data. Proper resistance (expressed by the inclination angle) is the maximum angle at which an individual can correctly perform the exercise. Resistance can be increased by adding one degree of inclination when an individual can complete 100 repetitions with correct movement in one session. Healthy individuals often use the 10 repetition maximum, but a more moderate load, such as the 20 repetition maximum or 30 repetition maximum, may be more suitable for elderly individuals or people with poor motivation.

A range of motion from 0 to 90° (or 60°) of flexion is frequently used in training with the sliding tilt table. Reducing the range of motion (i.e., decreasing the maximum flexion of joints) is necessary for individuals with joint pain or those who have difficulty extending flexed joints, especially for individuals with upper motor neuron lesions. Individuals with osteoarthritis may experience more pain with excessive joint flexion, so reducing the range of motion and increasing the inclination angle can allow them to exercise with the same intensity while minimizing joint pain. Decreasing the range of motion of hip and knee flexion also has two advantages for individuals with upper motor neuron lesions. First, it reduces the inhibitory effect of hip flexion on knee extensors in the affected lower extremity due to upper motor neuron lesions. Initially, hip joint flexion should be minimized in training with the sliding tilt table to avoid inhibiting knee extension. With improved motor control, the range of motion of the lower extremity joints can be increased. Second, it reduces the external load on body weight support muscles, making training easier, which is particularly important for people with severe motor impairment. One way to reduce the range of motion is to use an upward displacement of the bar that limits movement.

9.7.5.3 Correcting Hip External Rotation when Training with a Sliding Tilt Table

Many individuals with hemiparesis experience weakness in their hip internal rotators. It is common to observe people using the sliding tilt table with hip external rotation, but this is not the correct way to train, and it can become a bad habit. Thus, it is essential that this abnormal training be prevented.

Individuals should use their own hip internal rotators and maintain a neutral hip joint position in the transverse plane, thus avoiding external rotation, when training with the sliding tilt table.

They should control the external rotation of the hip joint using the internal rotators of the affected lower limb, rather than relying on manual assistance from others or using bandages to force the hip into a neutral position. These methods can potentially lead to learned nonuse of the hip internal rotator.

One effective approach is education. If individuals understand the importance of training in a neutral position in the transverse plane, they may correct their movement by themselves.

Sometimes, it may be necessary to decrease the inclination angle (or reduce the range of motion) to reduce the load on the affected lower extremity. This can make it easier for people to control hip external rotation with a reduced load on the affected lower limb.

9.7.5.4 Facilitate Lower Extremity Extension

Some people with gait disabilities are unable to extend their flexed lower extremity on the sliding tilt table in a low inclination angle. The initial approach for such people is always education. For individuals with aphasia, education can involve using body language and passive movement.

Providing assistance to individuals as they try to extend their flexed lower extremity can be helpful. Through this approach, individuals can learn how to use their own muscles to extend their affected lower extremity.

Practicing lower extremity extension with a healthcare provider in bed can also be beneficial. Initially, the healthcare provider can manually manipulate the hip and knee flexion in the affected lower limb while the individual is in a supine position, using one hand for support. Meanwhile, the other hand of the healthcare provider is placed on the sole of the affected limb, pressing on it, and the individual is asked to extend their flexed lower limb. If the individual cannot extend their flexed lower limb, passive extension can be used.

Additionally, reducing the training load by decreasing the inclination angle and range of motion can be helpful.

9.7.5.5 Facilitate Lower Extremity Flexion

In some cases, patients may be able to extend their lower limb from a flexed position but struggle to flex their lower limb from a fully extended position at the early stages of training. In such cases, asking individuals to extend their lower limb partially, rather than fully, can be helpful. It is generally easier to flex a lower limb from a partially flexed position than from a fully extended one. If this approach is not effective, manual assistance to flex the lower limb may be necessary.

9.7.5.6 Correcting Uncontrolled Flexion of the Lower Limb

Some individuals use the sliding tilt table while having uncontrolled flexion of the lower limb. Training eccentric contraction of the lower limb is important because many daily activities involve eccentric muscle contractions of the lower limb.

The primary method to correct uncontrolled flexion of the lower limb is through education. If individuals understand the importance of controlled flexion through education, they may be able to correct uncontrolled flexion on their own.

If education alone is not sufficient for proper training, it may be necessary to reduce the load by decreasing the inclination angle or range of motion.

9.7.5.7 Correcting Knee Hyperextension

Some individuals may use the sliding tilt table with knee hyperextension. However, practicing knee hyperextension while training on the sliding tilt table can lead to bad habits and walking with knee hyperextension.

The primary approach to correct knee hyperextension is education. If individuals continue to exhibit knee hyperextension despite education, other approaches may be necessary. Partially (not fully) extending the knee joint during training on the sliding tilt table can be beneficial as well.

9.7.5.8 Ensuring Full Range of Motion

Some individuals perform exercises with a partial range of motion when using the sliding tilt table. The target range of motion is typically set using a bar that restricts movement and is installed on the sliding tilt table. If individuals exercise with a partial range instead of the targeted range, the effectiveness of the training is reduced, and the number of repetitions becomes meaningless.

The initial approach to correction is education. If individuals understand the importance of training within the target range through education, they may be able to correct their errors during the training.

If education alone is not sufficient to lead proper training, it may be necessary to reduce the load by decreasing the inclination angle or range of motion.

9.7.5.9 Maintaining Heel Contact

Some individuals with ankle contractures cannot maintain heel contact with the footplate when their lower limb flexes. It is crucial to maintain heel contact during training with the sliding tilt table as maintaining contact with the entire foot is essential for proper standing and walking posture. Continuing training with a loss of heel contact can lead to it becoming a habit and may reduce postural stability during standing and walking. A short-term solution is to wear shoes with heels and toe-down rotation of the footplate to promote heel contact with the footplate. The long-term solution involves correcting ankle plantar flexion contractures, which will be detailed in a following chapter.

9.7.5.10 Training People with Wounds or Localized Pain

Training using the sliding tilt table is still possible for individuals with skin wounds or localized pain. This is because it is possible to prevent the wound or painful area from touching the sliding tilt table by placing a flat cushion or padding between the body and the sliding tilt table, leaving space for the wounded or painful area.

9.7.6 Training with Both Lower Limbs

9.7.6.1 Individuals with Lower Motor Neuron Lesion

Muscle strengthening requires training with appropriate resistance. For elderly individuals or those with gait disabilities, it may be suitable to exercise with moderate resistance, such as by targeting a specific number of repetitions, such as 20 repetitions maximum. Thirty repetitions maximum can be used for people with a poor health condition. Resistance can be increased by adjusting the inclination angle when individuals can perform more repetitions than the target number.

The amount of the load should be personalized based on the specific disease, the severity of impairment, and the individual's overall health condition.

9.7.6.2 Individuals with Upper Motor Neuron Lesion

People with hemiplegia must perform training with both lower limbs when using a sliding tilt table, training with the sliding tilt table offers these people various benefits. For instance, it provides weight-bearing to the hemiplegic lower limb and allows for passive motion of the hemiplegic lower limb using the unaffected lower limb. Additionally, it enables bilateral simultaneous muscle contraction during the initial stages of motor recovery. Since individuals with paralysis lack the muscle strength to control the external rotation of the hip joint on the hemiplegic side, it is necessary to use a bandage to control hip external rotation (Fig. 9.19). People with upper motor neuron lesion require many repetitions for strengthening, but there is no specific clinical data-based recommendation for the number of repetitions. One hundred times may be used as a tentative number of repetitions.

It is essential to exercise with an adequate inclination angle on the sliding tilt table to ensure

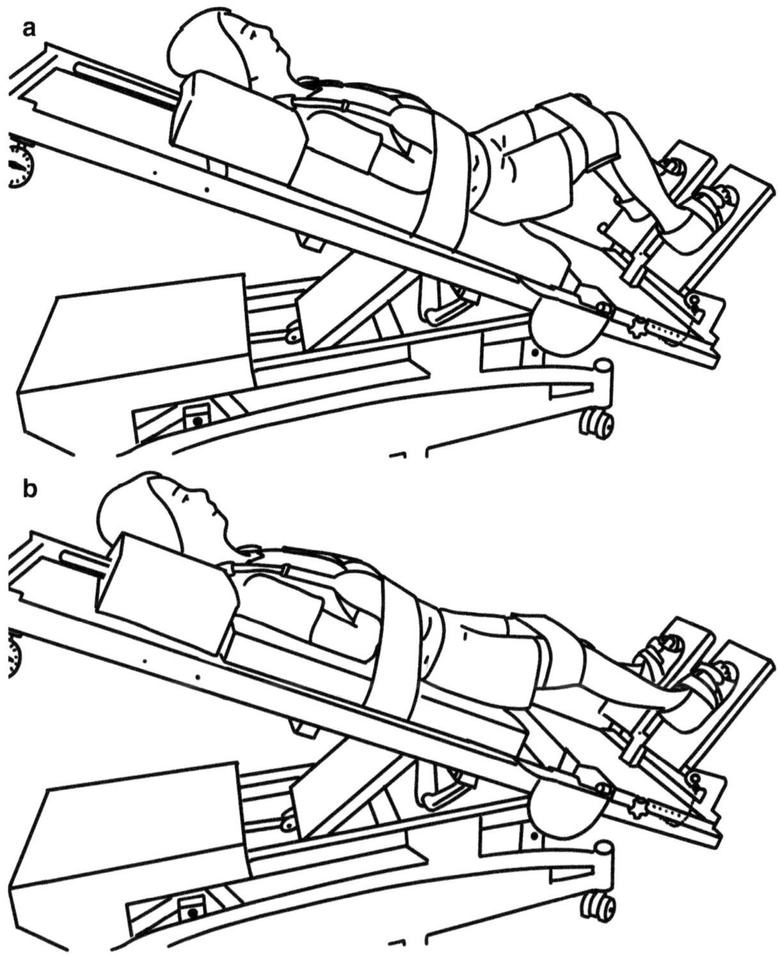

Fig. 9.19 Training with both lower limbs in people with hemiplegia. If one lower extremity is completely paralyzed, muscle contraction of the paralyzed lower extremity can be promoted by repeatedly pushing up the trunk using the opposite lower extremity while the paralyzed leg is underweight. (**a**) Starting position, (**b**) Final position

sufficient weight-bearing on the hemiplegic lower limb.

Some people with hemiplegia cannot exercise with a sufficient amount of inclination angle, which would be considered more than 20°, due to weakness of the unaffected lower limb. In such a case, decreasing the range of motion is a helpful way to make it possible for such subjects to exercise with proper weight-bearing.

9.7.7 Heel Lift Using a Sliding Tilt Table

9.7.7.1 Heel Lift Using a Single Lower Limb on a Sliding Tilt Table

Although ankle plantar flexors can be strengthened without a sliding tilt table, training with a sliding tilt table has several advantages (Fig. 9.20).

Because in the beginning, patients do not need to maintain balance when training using a sliding tilt table, it is very easy to perform strength training exercises. Secondly, the amount of resistance can be changed easily by changing the inclination angle of the sliding tilt table. So, people with severe muscle weakness (grade 2) can do muscle strengthening using heel lifts. Thirdly, feedback on the progress of strengthening is easy. Using the tilt angle and repetition numbers, patients can receive sensitive feedback on their progress, which can increase motivation for strengthening exercises.

The amount of load must be individualized according to the disease, severity of impairment, and general health condition. Strengthening for

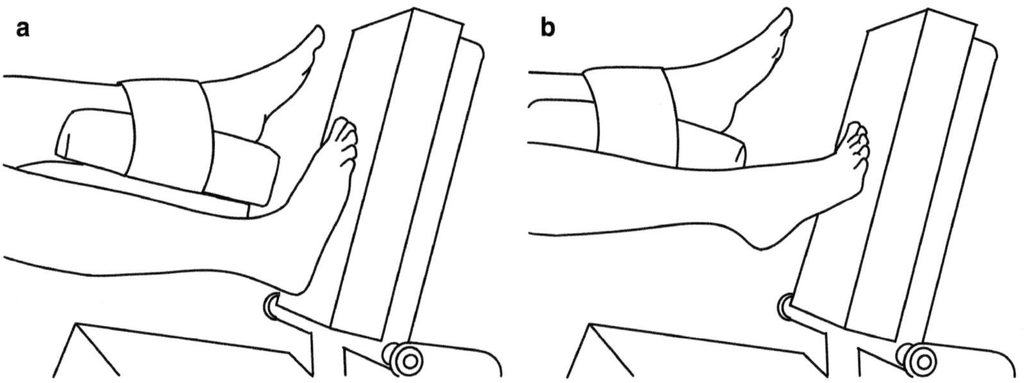

Fig. 9.20 Heel lift using a single lower limb on a sliding tilt table. If the affected plantar flexor muscles can produce a voluntary movement of the ankle joint, the affected plantar flexor muscles can be forced to use by placing the unaffected lower extremity on the leg raiser. (**a**) Starting position, (**b**) Final position

people with upper motor neuron lesions requires many repetitions; however, clinical data does not provide any recommendation for the amount of load. On a sliding tilt table, the resistance is determined by the inclination angle. Therefore, it is appropriate to adjust the inclination angle so that it is possible to lift the heel to a sufficient height more than 10 times. In healthy people, a 10-repetition maximum is frequently used. That said, more modest loads are suitable for elderly people or people with gait disabilities, such as through the use of a 20-repetition maximum.

For effective training, people must exercise using an adequate range of motion of the ankle joint. If the resistance is too high for people to perform the exercise, they may perform the movements with a limited range of motion. In such cases, it is necessary to decrease the inclination angle of the sliding tilt table.

Although some people have some muscle strength in ankle plantar flexors, they may not be able to lift their heel with minimal inclination angle. In that case, it is helpful for the healthcare provider to provide assistance when subjects make an effort to lift their heel. It may also be helpful to perform motor control training of the ankle plantar flexors in a supine position using manual resistance or an elastic band. Some people, especially those with upper motor neuron lesions, perform heel lifts with excessive inversion. In such cases, it is necessary to correct this abnormal performance using education or a reduction of resistance (i.e., inclination angle). Subjects may also find it beneficial to try to bear weight on the medial side of the foot.

9.7.7.2 Heel Lift Using Both Lower Limbs on a Sliding Tilt Table

For people with symmetric weakness, it is vital that they train with both lower limbs.

In people with symmetric lower limb weakness, a 10-repetition maximum can be used for relatively healthy people, and even with the elderly. However, more modest loads—such as a 20-repetition maximum—may be suitable for people with moderate or severe weakness. For effective training, people must exercise using an adequate range of motion of the ankle joint. If the resistance is too high for people to perform an exercise, they may perform the movement with a limited range of motion. In such cases, it is necessary to decrease the inclination angle of the sliding tilt table.

For people with no voluntary motion in ankle plantar flexor, it is mandatory to use both lower extremities to perform exercises on a sliding tilt table. It is also important that subjects exercise with a sufficient inclination angle of the sliding tilt table for adequate weight-bearing on the hemiplegic lower extremity. If people regain muscle strength in the affected lower extremity, training with both lower limbs must progress to training with a focus on the affected lower limb only.

9.8 Strengthening of Individual Muscles

When strengthening individual muscles, the training should be selective and correct. If muscle contraction occurs not only in the target muscle but also in nontargeted muscles, it may be harmful to functional recovery. This is more common in people with upper motor neuron lesions. To eliminate concurrent muscle contraction of nontargeted muscles, it is helpful to strengthen the targeted muscle with less effort to minimize the contraction of nontargeted muscles.

9.8.1 Back Extensors

While it is possible to strengthen the back extensor muscles in a prone position, it can be too difficult for many people with gait disabilities, and it may be inconvenient. Since resistance to back extensors is minimal in a nearly vertical sitting position, it is possible to strengthen the back extensors in people with severe weakness. That said, strengthening of the back extensors can be done while sitting through the use of two different methods.

One method involves isometric contractions. To perform this exercise, first, the subject must place their hands on a table, make an extension posture of the back, and maintain it for as long as possible. If the subject can maintain the extension posture for more than 1 min, they can progress to a more challenging task. Initially, subjects place their hands on a table, make an extension posture of the back, and then lift their hands from the table, striving to maintain this position for as long as possible. Although these methods may seem somewhat boring, they are very useful for people with back pain or for those who have undergone surgery. A less boring method is dynamic training, which involves reaching forward. People place their hands on a table or hospital bed in a trunk extension position, perform forward movements of the trunk and hands as far as possible, and then return to the starting position (Fig. 9.21). They repeat this forward and return movement as many times as possible.

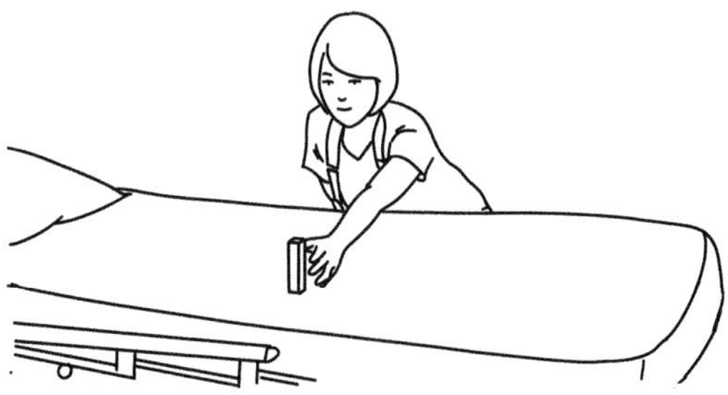

Fig. 9.21 Forward reaching with a hand on a hospital bed

If subjects regain muscle strength in the back extensors, they can perform this exercise with their hands in the air (Fig. 9.22).

A more exciting training method involves using an elastic band. After adjusting the length of the elastic band, subjects hold either end of the band with each hand in a sitting position. They then pull the elastic band as far as possible while maintaining a back extension posture. Lifting their hands above ear level is a helpful method to maintain back extension (Fig. 9.23).

After returning to the starting position, they repeat the pulling motion. As the strength of the back extensors increases, resistance can be increased by changing the distance of the pulling motion or by using an elastic band with more resistance.

9.8.2 Hip Flexors

For individuals with a muscle strength of grade 2, it is necessary to train in a posture that minimizes the effect of gravity, such as in the side-lying position or supine posture. Although the effect of gravity minimization is greater in the side-lying posture than in the supine posture, the supine posture is more stable and comfortable. It is preferable for people to exercise in the supine posture. At first, it may be helpful to provide external support to achieve a partially flexed position of the hip and knee joint (Fig. 9.24).

As strength in the hip flexor muscles is regained, training can progress to exercises without passive hip and knee flexion, starting from a hip and knee extension state (Fig. 9.25).

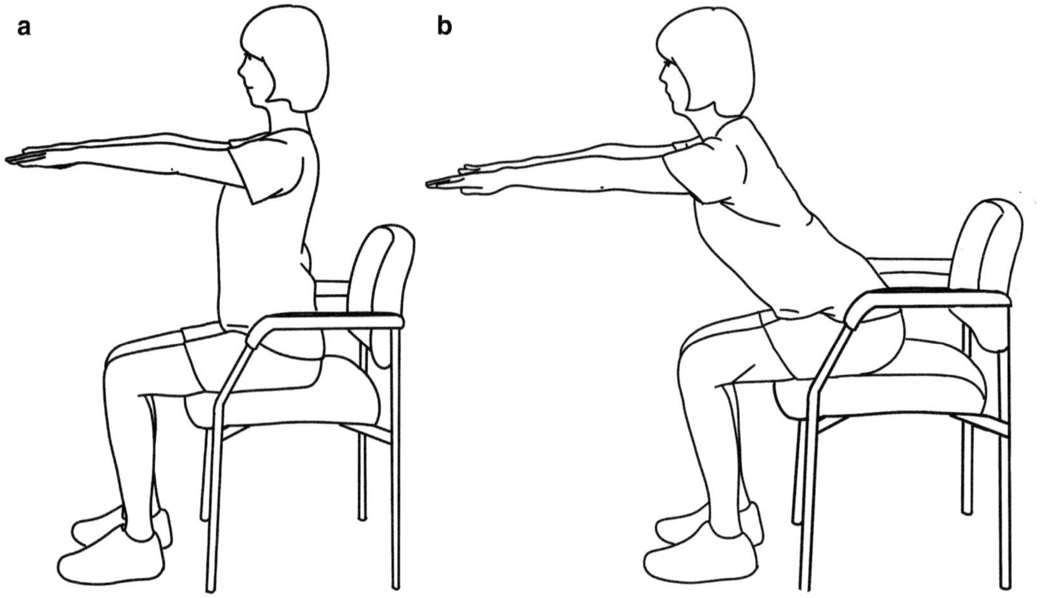

Fig. 9.22 Forward reaching with hands in the air. Forward reaching without touching the support surface is more difficult and more effective in strengthening the muscle strength of the trunk extension than forward reaching with touching the support surface. (**a**) Starting position, (**b**) Final position

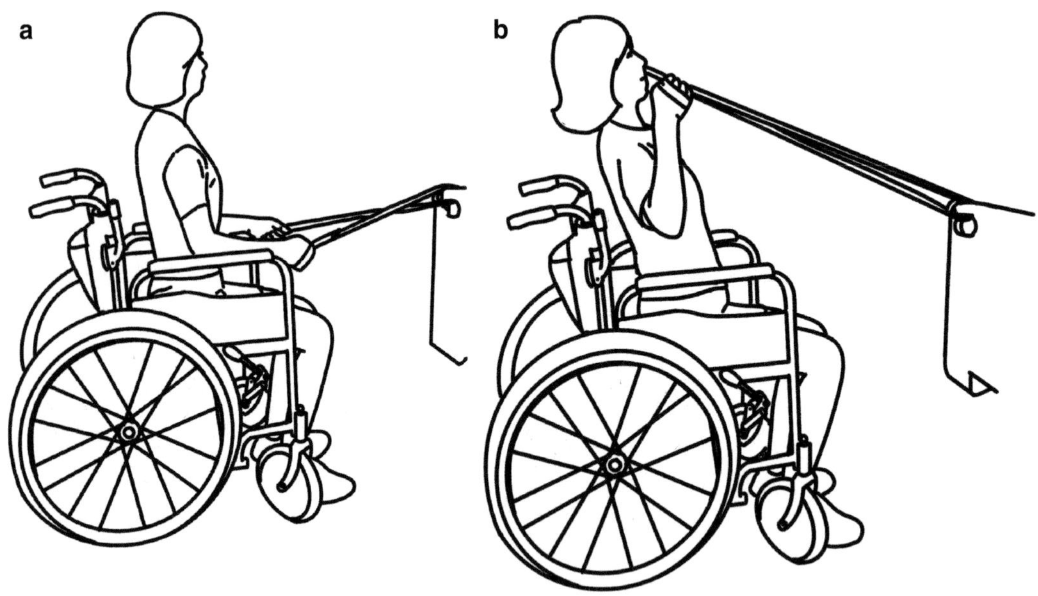

Fig. 9.23 Back extensor strengthening using an elastic band. It is possible to strengthen the strength of the trunk extension muscle using the rubber band fixed to the hospital bed. It is possible to promote trunk extension by moving the hands above the ear level. (**a**) Starting position, (**b**) Final position

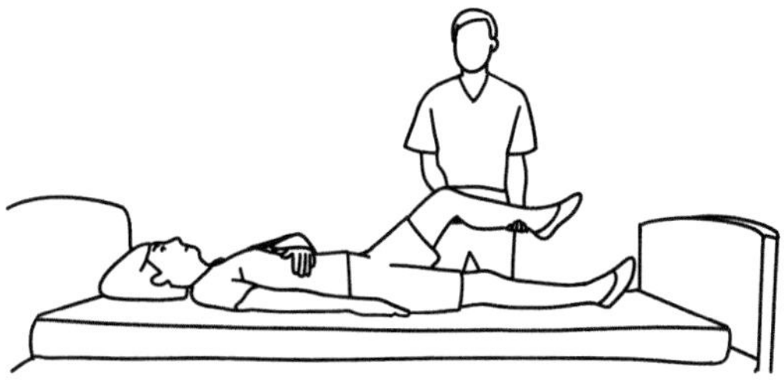

Fig. 9.24 Hip flexor strengthening with hip and knee flexion

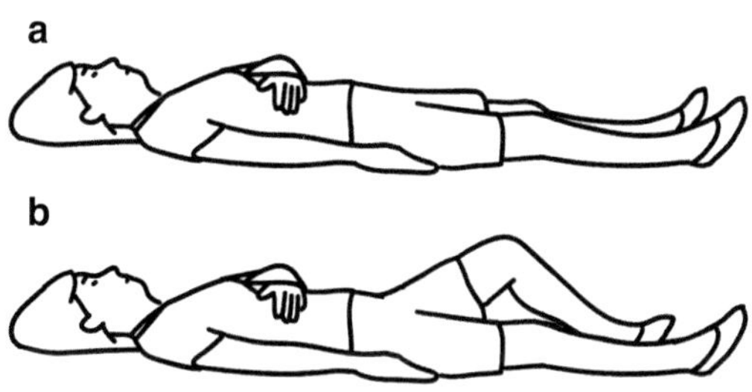

Fig. 9.25 Hip flexor strengthening in supine position. The strength of the hip flexor muscles can be increased by flexing the hip joint in a supine position while the legs are straight. (**a**) Starting position, (**b**) Final position

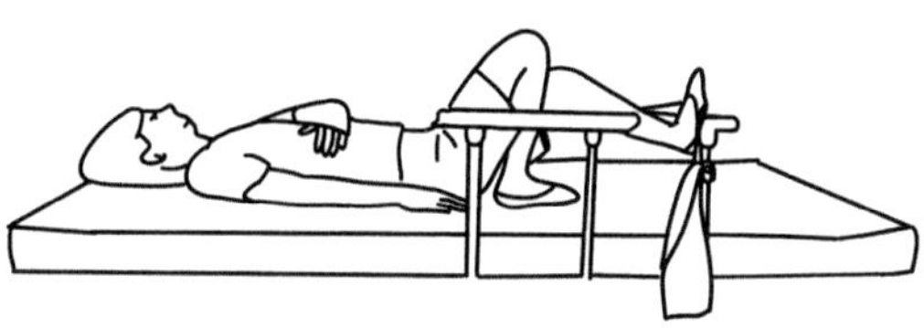

Fig. 9.26 Assistance of hip flexion through the use of the elastic recoil of a stretched elastic band

It is important to conduct training while maintaining a neutral position of the hip joint in the transverse plane, avoiding external rotation. In fact, hip flexion while maintaining a neutral position of the hip joint can strengthen the hip internal rotator. However, some people cannot maintain a neutral position of the hip joint during hip flexion, a problem that is more common in people with upper motor neuron lesions. In such cases, it is necessary to strengthen the hip internal rotators before training the hip flexors. Alternatively, training can be done in a side-lying posture. Elastic bands can assist with hip flexion in the supine position (Fig. 9.26).

If a patient cannot flex their hip in the supine position, they need to train in a side-lying position.

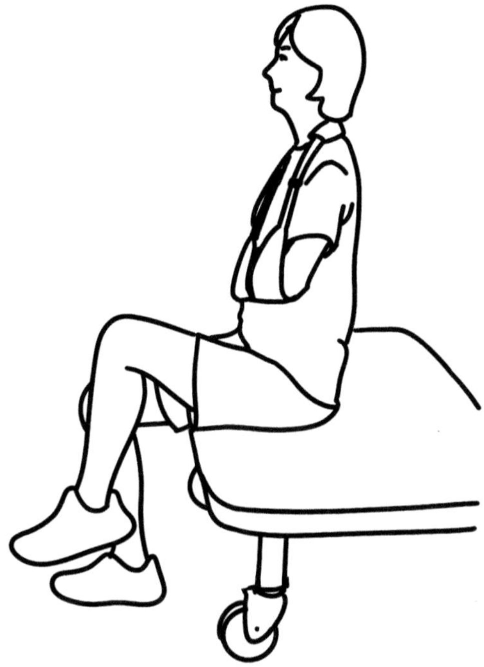

Fig. 9.27 Hip flexor strengthening in a sitting position

For people with muscle strength of grade 3 minus, it is possible to train in a sitting posture (Fig. 9.27).

Holding onto the armrest of a wheelchair or chair may be helpful as it increases postural stability. Like in training in the supine position, it is important to perform hip flexion while maintaining a neutral position of the hip joint in the transverse plane, avoiding hip external rotation. If this is not possible, it is necessary to decrease effort. Additionally, strengthening of the internal rotators of the hip joint is necessary.

For individuals with muscle strength of grade 3 or 4, it is possible to further strengthen using resistance, such as with an elastic band. The muscle strength of hip flexion can be increased using fast hip flexion, which may be helpful for further muscle strengthening.

9.8.3 Hip Extensors

Muscle Strength of Grade 0 or 1: Functional electrical stimulation can be used to strengthen the hip extensor. Training with a sliding tilt table is also a very effective method to strengthen the hip

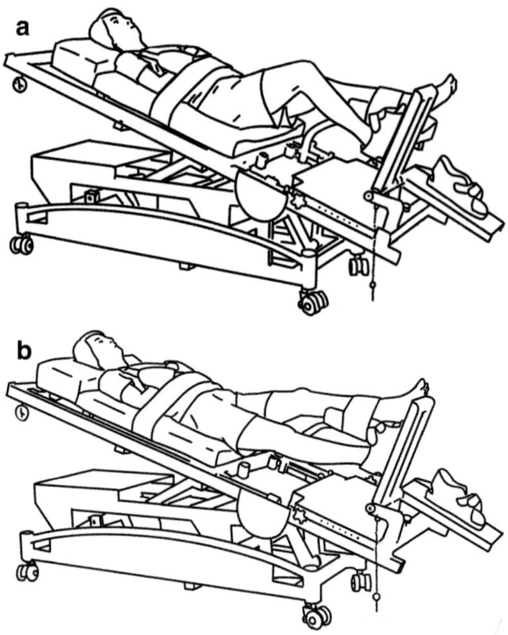

Fig. 9.28 Hip extensor strengthening with a sliding tilt table. Pushing up the trunk using the affected lower extremity on the sliding tilt table can strengthen the strength of the lower extremity extensor muscles (especially the hip and knee extensor muscles). (**a**) Starting position, (**b**) Final position

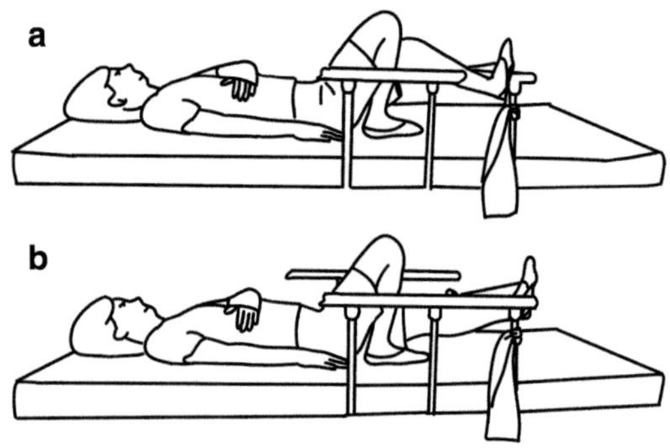

Fig. 9.29 Hip extensor strengthening with an elastic band. Pushing the rubber band fixed to the safety bars can strengthen the strength of the hip extension muscles. (**a**) Starting position, (**b**) Final position

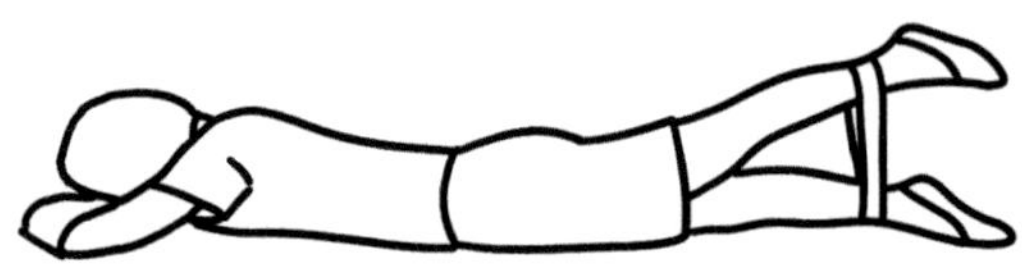

Fig. 9.30 Hip extensor strengthening with an elastic band

extensor. It makes it possible to bear weight on the affected lower limb, provides passive motion of the affected lower limb using the unaffected lower limb, and offers bilateral simultaneous contraction of the hip extensor muscles during the initial stages of motor recovery.

Muscle Strength of Grade 2: To minimize the effect of gravity, the side-lying position is widely used. To exercise in a side-lying posture, it is necessary to support the affected limb with a sling or the hand of a healthcare provider. However, this posture may not be comfortable. Training with a sliding tilt table is a very effective method to strengthen the hip extensor as it provides postural stability and quantitative data regarding resistance (Fig. 9.28).

Although a sliding tilt table allows for the easy changing of resistance, this equipment requires space and can be somewhat expensive to purchase, making it more suitable for clinics or hospitals.

Using an elastic band is a simpler way to strengthen the hip extensor in a supine position (Fig. 9.29).

Resistance can be increased by increasing the length of the elastic band or by switching to a stronger elastic band.

For individuals with a muscle strength of grade 3-, it is possible to perform strengthening exercises in the prone position. However, this posture may not be comfortable. Thus, strengthening with a sliding tilt table or elastic band is a more comfortable alternative.

For individuals with a muscle strength of grade 3 or 4, it is possible to strengthen the hip extensor through the use of bridging using one leg or both legs, depending on the subject's strength. An elastic band can also be used for hip extensor strengthening (Fig. 9.30).

Although bridging and elastic bands are effective methods for strengthening the hip extensor, training with a sliding tilt table is superior due to reasons mentioned before.

9.8.4 Hip Abductors

One important thing to understand about strengthening the hip abductors is the relationship between hip external rotation and hip abduction.

Since external rotation of the hip joint can cause the hip flexor to abduct the femur, preventing hip external rotation is essential for strengthening the hip abductor.

Muscle Strength of Grade 2: To train the hip abductors when a subject's muscle strength is at grade 2, it is necessary to use gravity-minimized postures, such as the supine posture or a standing posture. In the supine position, friction between the supporting surface and the body can interfere with hip abduction, so methods to reduce friction need to be employed. Placing the affected limb on a swing is an effective method to reduce friction. Alternatively, a slippery cloth or plate can be used. When performing hip abductor strengthening in a standing position, holding onto a safety bar can be helpful to increase postural stability. However, it is important to note that standing can be too difficult for many people with gait disabilities.

Muscle Strength of Grade 3-: After achieving a muscle strength of grade 3-, it is possible to further strengthen the hip abductors in the supine or side-lying position. The supine posture is preferred as it offers greater stability and comfort compared to the side-lying position. In the supine position, hip abductor training can be conducted using an elastic band.

Muscle Strength of Grade 3 or 4: After achieving a muscle strength of grade 3, it is possible to further strengthen the hip abductors using resistance, such as through the use of an elastic band (Fig. 9.31).

The muscle power of the hip abductors can be increased by performing fast hip abduction movements in a side-lying posture, which may be helpful for further muscle strengthening of the hip abductors.

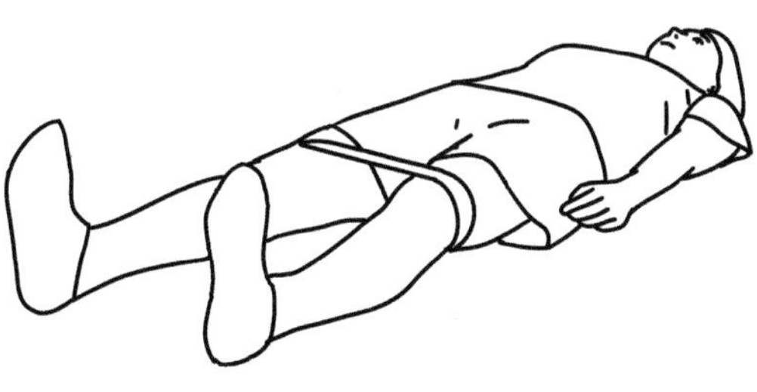

Fig. 9.31 Hip abductor strengthening with an elastic band

9.8.5 Hip Internal Rotators

Muscle Strength of Grade 2 minus: When strengthening the hip internal rotator in people with a muscle strength of grade 2 minus, the supine position is the optimal posture as it minimizes the effects of gravity. During training, individuals should have their hip and knee joints flexed, with the entire sole of the foot in contact with the supporting surface (Fig. 9.32).

To minimize the impact of gravity, it is important to control the amount of hip external rotation in the supine position. This can be achieved by adjusting the distance between the body and a nearby wall or side rail of a hospital bed. If the pelvis makes contact with the wall or rail, there is very little room for external rotation of the hip joint. As strength is regained, resistance can be increased by creating more distance between the body and the wall. An alternative method for training the hip internal rotator in the supine position is through the use of a loop elastic band fixed to a side rail. Such a band can be used to control the amount of hip internal rotation, progressing

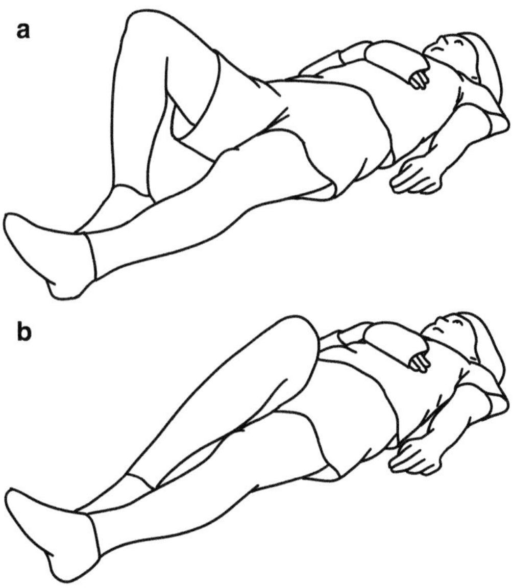

Fig. 9.32 Hip internal rotator strengthening in a supine position. The muscle strength of the internal rotational muscles of the hip joint can be strengthened by turning the affected knee inward in a supine position while bending and raising the affected knee. (**a**) Starting position, (**b**) Final position

from a partial hip internal rotation state to a no hip internal rotation state.

Some patients may have difficulty internally rotating the hip joint in positions where gravity is minimized or assisted. In such cases, facilitation methods may be necessary. These methods can include maintaining a neutral position of the contralateral hip in the transverse plane with hip and knee flexion, and contracting the affected hip internal rotator or simultaneous contraction of both hip internal rotators (Fig. 9.33).

If these methods are ineffective, forceful contraction of the contralateral hip internal rotator against resistance may help facilitate internal rotation of the affected hip.

Training in a partial side-lying position (i.e., rotating the body approximately 45° with the affected side facing up) is another option, with the use of a pillow or balloon placed between the legs to maintain the proper position. Start with slight internal rotation of the hip joint, and by contracting the hip internal rotator, this leads to more internal rotation of the hip joint. To prevent sliding down (passive extension of the hip and knee joint), it may be necessary to hold the foot or distal tibia while using their unaffected lower limb to support the affected lower limb (Fig. 9.34).

As muscle strength increases, training can progress without the need for facilitation methods, and resistance against hip internal rotation can be increased by adjusting the distance between the body and the wall.

Muscle Strength of Grade 2: For individuals with a muscle strength of grade 2, strengthening can be performed in a sitting position. Initially, they can sit in a wheelchair and place their feet on the footplate, and then contract the affected hip internal rotator without contracting the unaffected hip internal rotator. While maintaining this position, it is preferable for the thigh not to make contact with the seat of the wheelchair so as to reduce friction (Fig. 9.35).

Muscle Strength of Grade 3 or 4: After achieving a muscle strength of grade 3, further strengthening can be accomplished using resistance, such as an elastic band (Fig. 9.36).

Bridging with one leg may also be beneficial for strengthening the hip internal rotator. If bridging with one leg proves to be too difficult, it may be necessary to modify the exercise method. One approach is to start with bridging while using both legs, and then lift the unaffected lower limb and maintain that posture before returning to the starting position. This sequence can be repeated for further strengthening.

a

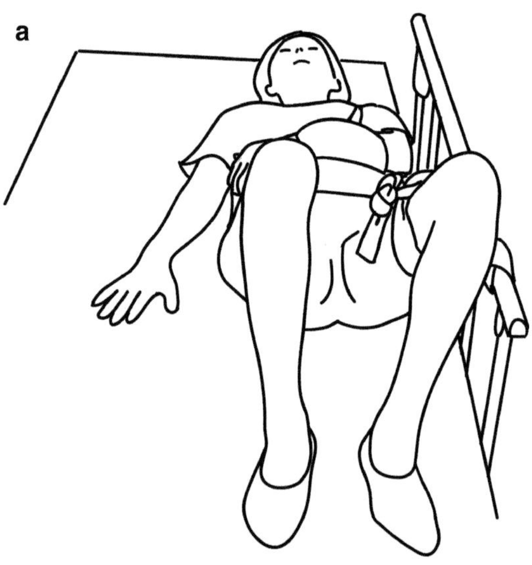

b

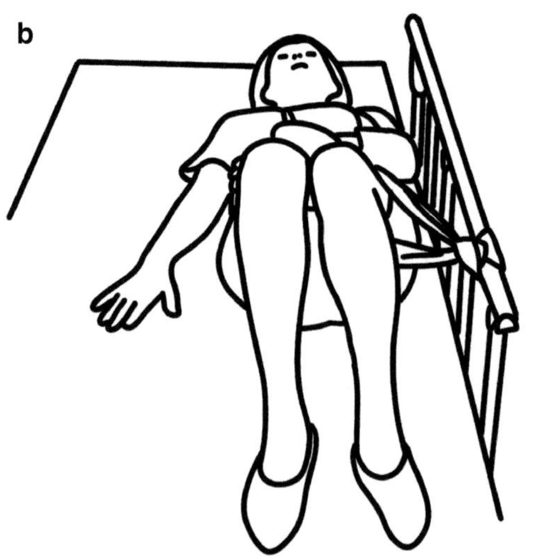

Fig. 9.33 Hip internal rotator strengthening using co-contraction of the contralateral hip internal rotator. The contraction of the hip internal rotator of the opposite hip may facilitate the contraction of the internal rotator of the affected hip. (**a**) Starting position, (**b**) Final position

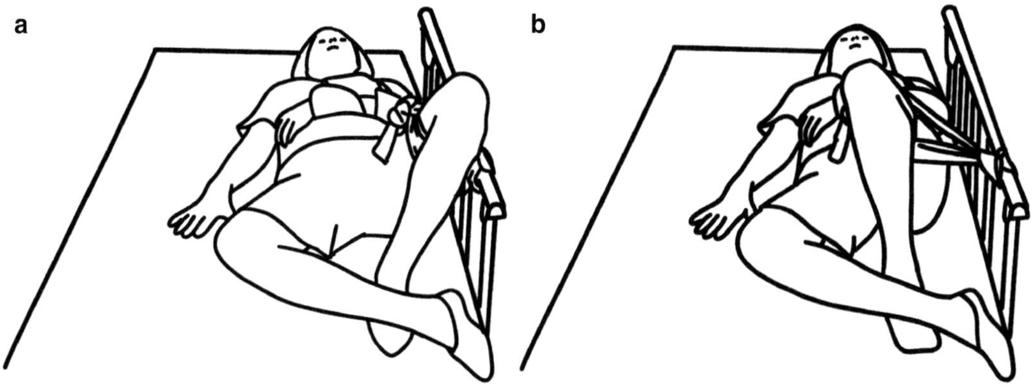

Fig. 9.34 Hold the affected foot during hip internal rotator strengthening. If the affected lower extremity is extended spontaneous during the strengthening of hip internal rotator, extension of affected lower extremity can be prevented by using the opposite lower extremity. (**a**) Starting position, (**b**) Final position

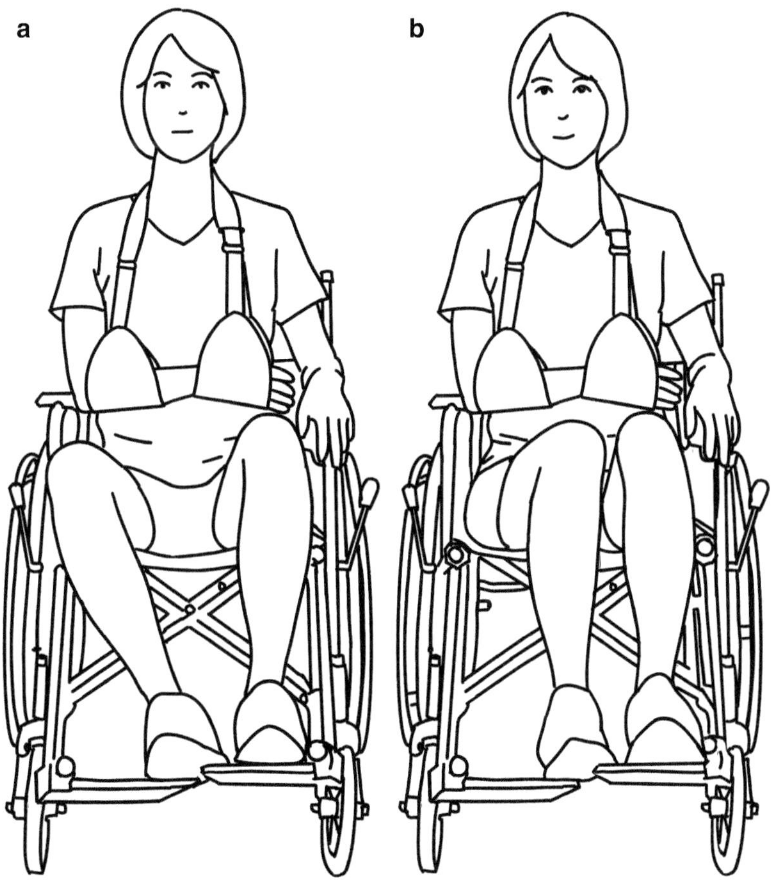

Fig. 9.35 Hip internal rotator strengthening in a sitting position. (**a**) Starting position, (**b**) Final position

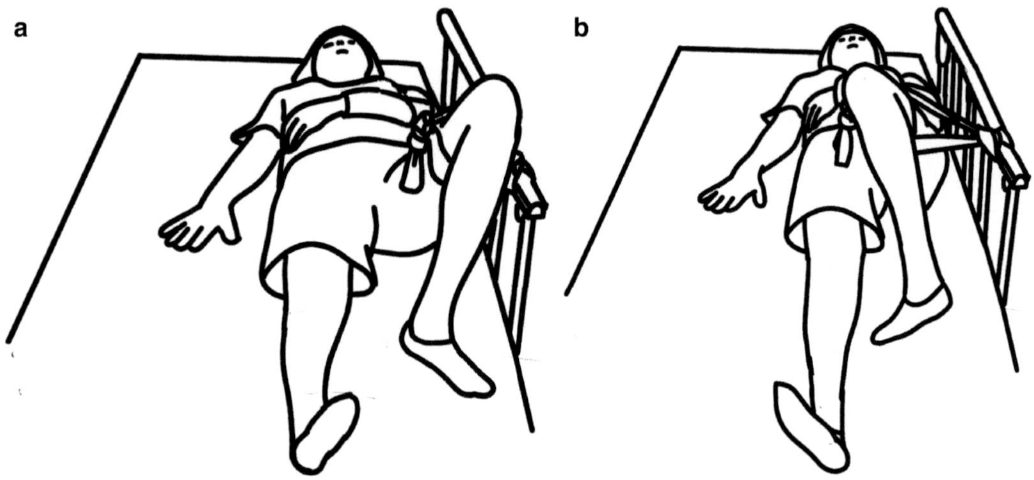

Fig. 9.36 Hip internal rotator strengthening using an elastic band. Muscle strength can be performed more effectively by applying resistance to the hip internal rotator using a rubber band fixed to the safety bar. (**a**) Starting position, (**b**) Final position

9.8.6 Knee Extensor Strengthening

For individuals with a muscle strength of grade 0 or 1 in the knee extensor, functional electrical stimulation can be utilized as a method to strengthen the knee extensor muscles. Training with a sliding tilt table is also highly effective for this purpose. This approach allows for weight-bearing on the affected lower limb, passive motion of the affected lower limb assisted by the unaffected lower limb, and also has the added benefit of bilateral simultaneous contraction of the knee extensor muscles during the initial stages of motor recovery.

For individuals with a muscle strength of grade 2 in the knee extensor, training in a gravity-minimized posture is recommended, and this can be achieved in the side-lying position. However, in the side-lying position, friction between the supporting surface and the body can hinder knee extension. To address this, methods to reduce friction should be employed, such as placing the affected limb on a swing. Another effective method for strengthening the knee extensor is training with a sliding tilt table, which provides postural stability and allows for easy the adjustment of resistance.

Functional electrical stimulation can also be used as a method to strengthen the knee extensor in individuals with grade 2 muscle strength.

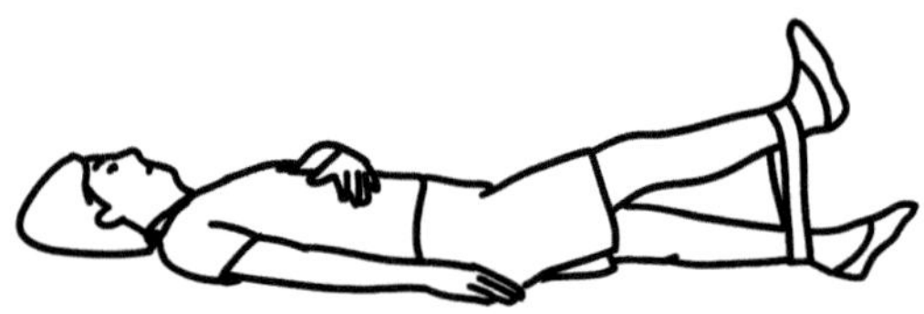

Fig. 9.37 Knee extensor strengthening with an elastic band

Individuals with a muscle strength of grade 3- can perform knee extensor strengthening exercises in a sitting position. They can start by sitting on the edge of a hospital bed and contracting the knee extensor as strongly as possible. Training with a sliding tilt table remains a highly effective method for strengthening the knee extensor in individuals with muscle strength at this level.

For those with a muscle strength of grade 3 or 4 in the knee extensor, a different method can be employed using an elastic band. In this case, individuals should lie down with their back on a supporting surface with an elastic band wrapped around both ankles. While maintaining knee extension, they should flex the hip joint of the affected lower limb as strongly as possible against the resistance of the elastic band. To prevent passive lifting of the unaffected lower limb, it may be necessary to contract the hip extensor of the unaffected lower limb (Fig. 9.37). This exercise method is a particularly useful method when there is arthritis in the knee joint.

Training with an elastic band is effective for strengthening the knee extensor, but it should be noted that exercises like the sit-to-stand or squatting with a chair are less boring methods to achieve knee extensor strengthening.

9.8.7 Ankle Dorsiflexor Strengthening

In the strengthening of the ankle dorsiflexor, hip and knee flexion play important roles. Initially, a knee-flexed posture can help loosen the gastrocnemius muscle, and hip flexion can inhibit the extension synergy of the lower limb, making ankle dorsiflexion easier.

For individuals with a muscle strength of grade 0 or 1 in the ankle dorsiflexor, functional electrical stimulation can be used to strengthen this muscle group. Additionally, forceful contraction of the hip flexors against resistance may facilitate the contraction of the ankle dorsiflexors.

For individuals with a muscle strength of grade 2, functional electrical stimulation remains a viable method for strengthening the ankle dorsiflexors. Strengthening exercises can be performed in a supine or side-lying position with hip and knee flexion. In addition, the elastic recoil of an elastic band can be utilized to assist with ankle dorsiflexion (Fig. 9.38).

Muscle Strength of Grade 3-: Individuals with a muscle strength of grade 3- can perform ankle dorsiflexor strengthening exercises in a sitting position. Sitting on the edge of a hospital bed and contracting the ankle dorsiflexor as strongly as possible is recommended. Holding onto the side rail of the hospital bed can also help increase postural stability.

Muscle Strength of Grade 3 or 4: After achieving a muscle strength of grade 3, further strengthening of the ankle dorsiflexors can be accomplished using resistance, such as with the use of an elastic band. Muscle power of the ankle dorsiflexors can be increased by performing fast ankle dorsiflexion exercises, which can aid in further muscle strengthening.

9.8.8 Ankle Plantar Flexor Strengthening

Muscle Strength of Grade 0 or 1: Functional electrical stimulation can be used to strengthen the ankle plantar flexor in individuals with a muscle strength of grade 0 or 1. Additionally, training with a sliding tilt table is highly effective as it enables weight-bearing on the affected lower limb, provides passive motion assisted by the unaffected lower limb, and allows for bilateral simultaneous contraction of the ankle plantar flexor muscles during the initial stages of motor recovery.

Muscle Strength of Grade 2: For individuals with a muscle strength of grade 2, it is important to train in a gravity-minimized posture, such as while lying in the supine position. Manual resistance in the supine position can be used to strengthen the ankle plantar flexor, with the resistance level increasing as muscle strength improves. Using an elastic band can also be a useful method for strengthening the ankle plantar flexor in the supine position (Fig. 9.39).

Additionally, hip and knee extension can be helpful, as ankle plantar flexion is a component of the extension synergy. Resistance should be progressively increased as training progresses.

Individuals with a muscle strength of grade 2 plus can perform ankle plantar flexor strengthen-

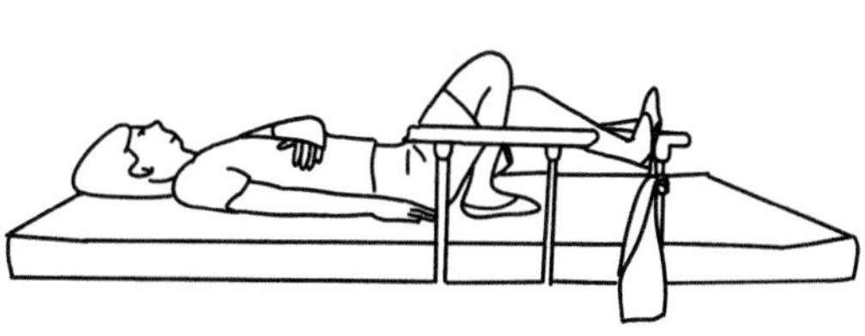

Fig. 9.38 Ankle dorsiflexor strengthening using the assistance of an elastic recoil

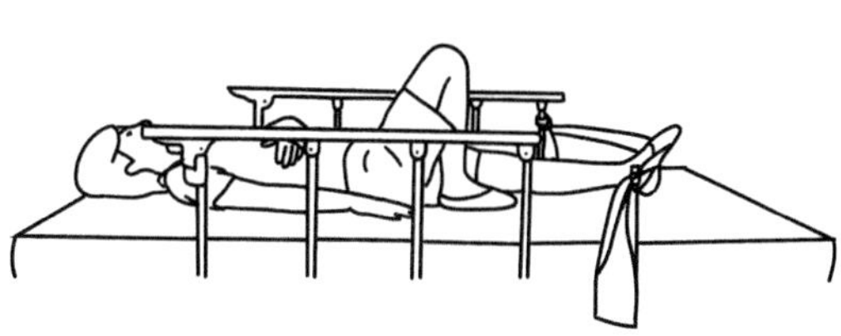

Fig. 9.39 Ankle plantar flexor strengthening using an elastic band

ing exercises in a standing position using both lower limbs. However, performing a heel lift with both limbs can lead to learned non-use of the affected lower limb in people with upper motor neuron lesions. To prevent learned nonuse of the affected lower limb, forced use of the affected limb can be achieved using a chair or step. This concept was previously mentioned in the Sect. 9.5.

Muscle Strength of Grade 3-: Individuals with a muscle strength of grade 3- can perform ankle plantar flexor strengthening exercises in a standing position using only the affected lower limb. Training can be done while standing with hands resting on the wall and by lifting the affected heel as high as possible.

Muscle Strength of Grade 3 or 4: For individuals with a muscle strength of grade 3 or 4, ankle plantar flexor strengthening can be achieved using unilateral heel lifts. Further strengthening can be accomplished by increasing the speed of the heel lifts and the number of repetitions. Training with a sliding tilt table remains an effective method for strengthening the ankle plantar flexors, and muscle power can be increased by performing fast heel lifts.

9.9 Power Training

Power is needed for increased mobility and regaining balance. Before power training, the strength of antigravity muscles should be regained. Body weight support muscles can be trained using hopping. For safety, keeping contact with the wall using both hands is recommended at the initial stage of training. It should be noted that this form of training may be harmful to people with osteoporosis or musculoskeletal problems. The power of the ankle plantar flexor can be trained using a sliding tilt table (Fig. 9.40).

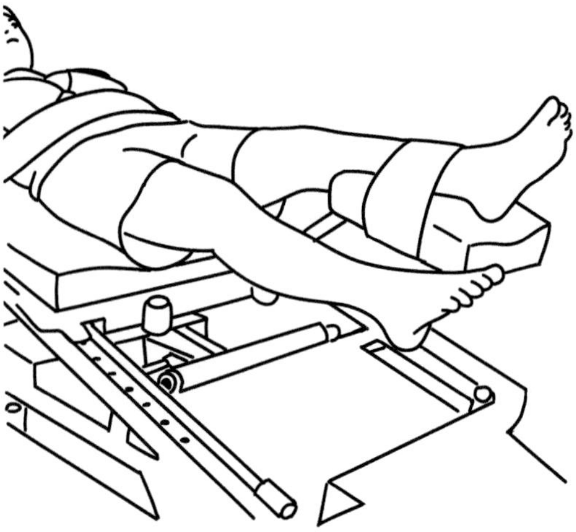

Fig. 9.40 Power training of the ankle plantar flexor using a sliding tilt table

9.10 Summary

The recovery of strength in patients with upper motor neuron lesions is achieved through several mechanisms, including diaschisis, disinhibition, and plastic changes in synapses. Among these mechanisms, changes in synapses are the most important for regaining muscle strength induced by training. Achieving changes in synapses requires numerous repetitions.

Effective strengthening relies on using an appropriate amount of resistance, and determining this through repetition numbers is more convenient than simply relying on the percentage of a one-repetition maximum.

When selecting resistance for strengthening in people with upper motor neuron lesions, it is imperative to ensure that it does not lead to incorrect movements, such as unnecessary associated movements or uncontrolled contractions.

Weight-bearing on the lower limb stimulates Golgi's tendon organs, skin somatosensory receptors, and muscle spindles. Consequently, it promotes the contraction of body weight support muscles.

Exercise within a closed kinetic chain is widely used in sports rehabilitation and gait training. It offers several advantages for strengthening body weight support muscles, including the ability to strengthen multiple muscles simultaneously and train multi-joint coordination. In addition, it is more functional as body weight support muscles work in a closed kinetic chain during gait. Furthermore, this type of training does not require special equipment.

Postural stability is crucial for successful strengthening exercises. Therefore, exercises performed in a lying-down position are particularly beneficial for individuals with balance issues or upper motor neuron lesions.

References

Ada L, Dorsch S, Canning CG. Strengthening interventions increase strength and improve activity after stroke: a systematic review. Aust J Physiother. 2006;52(4):241–8.

Awad LN, Binder-Macleod SA, Pohlig RT, Reisman DS. Paretic propulsion and trailing limb angle are key determinants of long-distance walking function after stroke. Neurorehabil Neural Repair. 2015;29(6):499–508.

Borde R, Hortobágyi T, Granacher U. Dose-dose response relationships of resistance training in healthy old adults: a systematic review and meta-analysis. Sports Med. 2015;45(12):1693–720.

Buchner DM, Larson EB, Wagner EH, Koepsell TD, de Lateur BJ. Evidence for a non-linear relationship between leg strength and gait speed. Age Ageing. 1996;25(5):386–91.

Cheng PT, Chen CL, Wang CM, Hong WH. Leg muscle activation patterns of sit-to-stand movement in stroke patients. Am J Phys Med Rehabil. 2004;83(1): 10–6.

Duncan P, Studenski S, Richards L, Gollub S, Lai SM, Reker D, Perera S, Yates J, Koch V, Rigler S, Johnson D. Randomized clinical trial of therapeutic exercise in subacute stroke. Stroke. 2003;34(9): 2173–80.

Duysens J, Clarac F, Cruse H. Load-regulating mechanisms in gait and posture: comparative aspects. Physiol Rev. 2000;80(1):83–133.

Flanagan S, Salem GJ, Wang MY, Sanker SE, Greendale GA. Squatting exercises in older adults: kinematic and kinetic comparisons. Med Sci Sports Exerc. 2003;35(4):635–43.

Judge JO, Underwood M, Gennosa T. Exercise to improve gait velocity in older persons. Arch Phys Med Rehabil. 1993;74(4):400–6.

Kesar TM, Perumal R, Reisman DS, Jancosko A, Rudolph KS, Higginson JS, Binder-Macleod SA. Functional electrical stimulation of ankle plantarflexor and dorsiflexor muscles: effects on poststroke gait. Stroke. 2009;40(12):3821–7.

Lewek MD, Schmit BD, Hornby TG, Dhaher YY. Hip joint position modulates volitional knee extensor muscle activity after stroke. Muscle Nerve. 2006;34(6):767–74.

Ouellette MM, LeBrasseur NK, Bean JF, Phillips E, Stein J, Frontera WR, Fielding RA. High-intensity resistance training improves muscle strength, self-reported function, and disability in long-term stroke survivors. Stroke. 2004;35(6):1404–9.

Rodosky MW, Andriacchi TP, Andersson GB. The influence of chair height on lower limb mechanics during rising. J Orthop Res. 1989;7(2):266–71.

Shumway-Cook A, Woollacott MH, Rachwani J, Santamaria V. Clinical management of the patient with a mobility disorder (Chapter 16). In: Motor control: translating research into clinical practice. 6th ed. Philadelphia: Lippincott Williams & Wilkins; 2023. p. 440–89.

Speirs DE, Bennett MA, Finn CV, Turner AP. Unilateral vs. bilateral squat training for strength, sprints, and agility in academy Rugby players. J Strength Condition Res. 2016;30(2):386–92.

Trees DW, Ketelsen CA, Hobbs JA. Use of a modified tilt table for preambulation strength training as an adjunct to burn rehabilitation: a case series. J Burn Care Rehabil. 2003;24(2):97–103.

van den Tillaar R, Larsen S. Kinematic and EMG comparison between variations of unilateral squats under different stabilities. Sports Med Int Open. 2020;4(2):E59–66.

Yang YR, Mi PL, Huang SF, Chiu SL, Liu YC, Wang RY. Effects of neuromuscular electrical stimulation on gait performance in chronic stroke with inadequate ankle control—A randomized controlled trial. PLoS One. 2018;13(12):e0208609.

Balance Training 10

10.1 Effectiveness of Balance Training

In many people with walking disabilities, the primary cause is a balance problem. The effectiveness of balance training has been confirmed by numerous clinical studies (Lesinski et al. 2015).

10.2 Principles of Balance Training

10.2.1 Safety

To make balance training effective, challenging balance tasks are necessary, but they come with a risk of falling. Thus, it is crucial to implement strategies to prevent falls during balance training. Various safety measures, such as using an overhead harness, having a healthcare provider present for support, and utilizing walls and chairs, have already been discussed in the chapter on balance evaluation. In balance training, another technique is to perform the task in a horizontally narrow space that can be used to prevent falls. Detailed information on narrowing the space will be provided in the section on one-leg squats.

10.2.2 Anxiety of Falling

If people are anxious about falling, they may not fully participate in challenging balance tasks. As such, it is necessary to reduce anxiety using helpful methods. Using a safety bar is not a good option because it causes people to become dependent on the use of their unaffected upper extremity. Instead, manual touch for individuals with balance problems may be helpful. Using a safety belt and having it held by a healthcare provider may help relieve anxiety. An overhead harness is the most effective means to prevent falls. Although there is nearly no risk of falling when using an overhead harness, people may still have a fear of falling when there is no tension in the harness. Demonstrating safety through planned falls when secured in the overhead harness system may be helpful in alleviating such anxiety.

10.2.3 Reduce the Base of Support

To make balance training effective, minimizing the area of the base of support and reducing hand usage is essential in order to improve balance (Allen et al. 2011). Using the hands to support one's balance extends the base of support and may lead to learned nonuse of the affected lower limb, potentially interfering with the recovery of normal gait. Therefore, hand usage should be minimized for effective balance training. While in the final stages of balance training, exercises should be performed without the use of hands, but in the initial stages, some individuals with balance problems may need to use their hands for balance.

Y.-S. Lee, *Task Oriented Gait Training*, https://doi.org/10.1007/978-981-97-3348-4_10

There is a hierarchy in hand usage for balance training. The heaviest hand usage involves holding onto a stable object, such as a stall bar or safety bar. Holding can be used to support body weight (i.e., control vertical movement) and manage horizontal movements of the body in all directions.

The next level involves propping against a support surface, such as a treatment table, with one's hands. This can help a person support their body weight and control horizontal movement of the body in one direction. If the body moves in the opposite direction of the prop, the prop cannot control horizontal movement. The use of walking aids, such as a cane or walker, has a similar effect. If people with balance problems have sufficient muscle strength to support their body weight, holding something or propping against something may not be necessary for supporting their body weight. The amount of hand usage needed to support body weight can be checked using a pressure sensor system.

One level up from this involves touching the wall with one's hands and leaning against it. Touching the wall cannot be used to support body weight; it can only control the horizontal movement of the body in one direction. Most of the time, people lean forward against a wall. To reduce the amount of leaning, it is helpful to ask people to shift their body weight toward their heels. If people tilt forward excessively, moving them back toward the wall can help. If people lean their back against the wall, asking them to shift their body weight toward their toes can reduce the amount of leaning.

Finally, the lightest hand usage involves touching the wall with just one's fingertips. The fingertips provide sensory input about the amount of leaning and can contribute to maintaining a standing posture. As balance training progresses, it is essential to reduce hand usage in the aforementioned order.

10.2.4 Movement of the Center of Mass

It is important to move the center of mass to improve balance (Allen et al. 2011). While horizontal movement is widely used in training, vertical movement is relatively less utilized. To enhance balance, it is necessary to move the center of mass not only horizontally but also vertically. It is possible to quantitatively assess the amount of vertical movement using changes in ground reaction force. Precise control of the movement of the center of mass is crucial. Training while placing a paper cup over one's head (or simply imagining placing a paper cup over one's head) can help refine the precise control of the center of mass movement (Fig. 10.1).

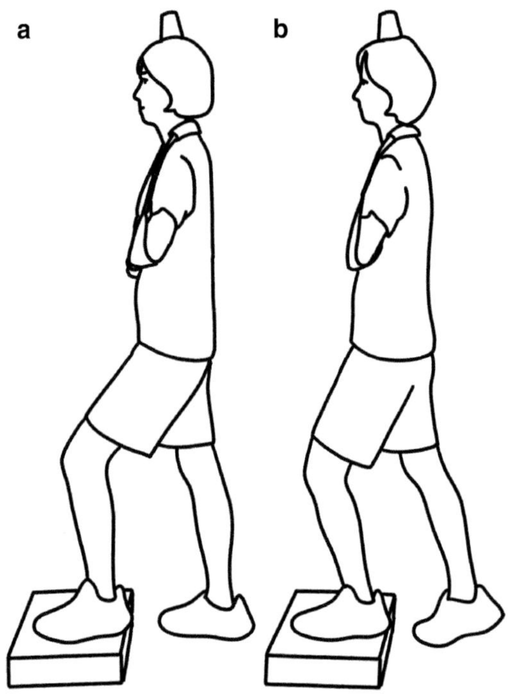

Fig. 10.1 Training the precise control of movement of the center of mass using a paper cup. Movement controlled to the point of not dropping the cup on the head while doing step-up is more effective in improving balance ability. (**a**) Starting position, (**b**) Final position

It is also possible to quantitatively assess the control of movement using the degree of smoothness and the amount of changes in ground reaction force.

10.2.5 Progressive Training

Effective balance training should challenge individuals with balance problems

(Sherrington et al. 2011). The difficulty of the task can be increased by reducing the base of support and sensory input (American College of Sports Medicine et al. 2009), increasing the magnitude of movement, increasing the requirement for precise control of movement, and introducing dual tasks. For older adults, moderate to highly challenging balance exercises are required to improve balance and reduce the risk of falling (Sherrington et al. 2011).

In normal development, toddlers gain steady-state balance first, followed by proactive balance, and finally reactive balance. Therefore, using the same sequence of balance training may be a good strategy for balance training.

10.3 Sitting Balance Training

10.3.1 Head Control Training

In a vertical position, the effect of gravity is minimized. Therefore, it is good to start head control training in a vertical position. If one's trunk balance is poor, individuals can sit in a wheelchair with their back in contact with the backrest. By using the backrest, people can concentrate on head control. Alternatively, sitting with arms placed on a lapboard may be helpful in maintaining a sitting position without leaning on the backrest. Changing from a supine position to sitting may also be helpful to improve alertness. Since individuals with impaired alertness may not report symptoms of orthostatic hypertension, checking the blood pressure before training in a sitting position is absolutely mandatory. To accomplish this, make the neck and head vertical using manual assistance. Then gradually decrease the assistance and have the individual maintain a vertical position. After the patient can maintain a vertical position on their own, have them slightly flex their neck and then return to a vertical position. Gradually increase the amount of flexion or extension and have them return to a vertical position.

10.3.2 Steady-State Balance Training

Many patients with severe motor impairment sit with their backs reclined against the backrest of a wheelchair. This sitting position may lead to learned nonuse of the trunk muscles. The first step in sitting balance training is to move the trunk forward. In patients with severe motor impairment, it is helpful to place their forearms on a table, bed, or lapboard. Training for sitting balance using a wheelchair and hospital bed has many advantages. For example, it does not require the purchase of new equipment and is considered very safe for people with balance problems.

The next step is to create lumbar lordosis by using the back extensor muscles while the forearms are placed on a table, bed, or lapboard. If the patient can maintain lumbar lordosis for 1 min, instruct them to lift both forearms in the air and gradually increase the time spent lifting them (Fig. 10.2).

Since this training minimizes stress on the back, it is very helpful for people with back pain. However, static training can be somewhat boring for individu-

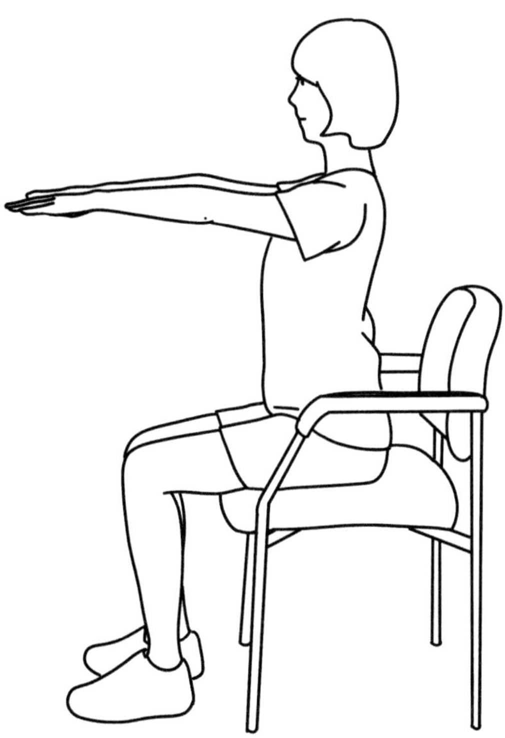

Fig. 10.2 Steady-state balance training

als with balance problems, so it can become difficult for them to concentrate on the training.

10.3.3 Proactive Balance Training

More dynamic training in people with severe balance problems can be accomplished by having the subjects reach forward and then return to the starting position while their hands are on top of a therapeutic ball, table, bed, or lapboard. With sufficient improvement of their sitting balance, this action can be done with one's hands in the air (Fig. 10.3).

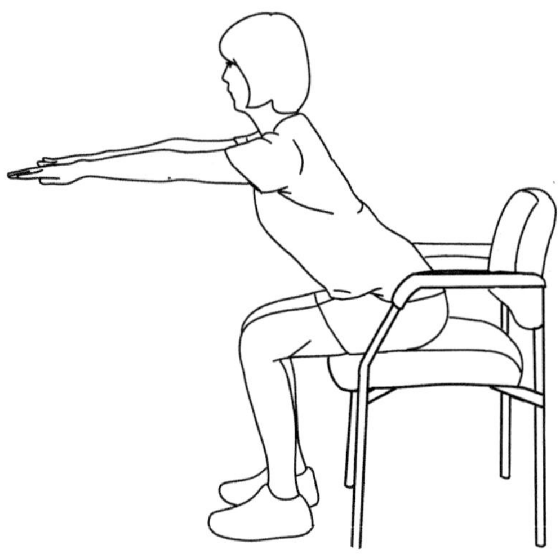

Fig. 10.3 Forward reaching with hands in the air

Reaching with a therapeutic ball is a popular method for training to improve sitting balance. However, reaching with a bed or mat offers several advantages over using a therapeutic ball. Another benefit is that it does not require additional equipment as most people or hospitals already have a bed or mat. Additionally, this sort of training is safer and more comfortable for people with balance problems because the bed or mat provides more stable support. Placing a paper cup on top of the bed or mat can act as a target and may be helpful for training (Fig. 10.4).

In forward reach training, it is important for the feet to be placed on the floor rather than on a footrest. This position facilitates weight-bearing on the feet and forward movement of the trunk. Different directions can be used for reaching, including straight forward, diagonal right forward, diagonal left forward, left lateral, and right lateral.

This training is simpler and more interesting for people with balance problems compared to static balance training. It is also suitable for individuals with poor cognition. As balance improves, the training can progress to include a larger range of movement and training while keeping the hands in the air.

Some patients may exhibit lateral instability and tilt to one side of the body. In such cases, reaching to the opposite side with a hand on the top of the table can be beneficial. External sup-

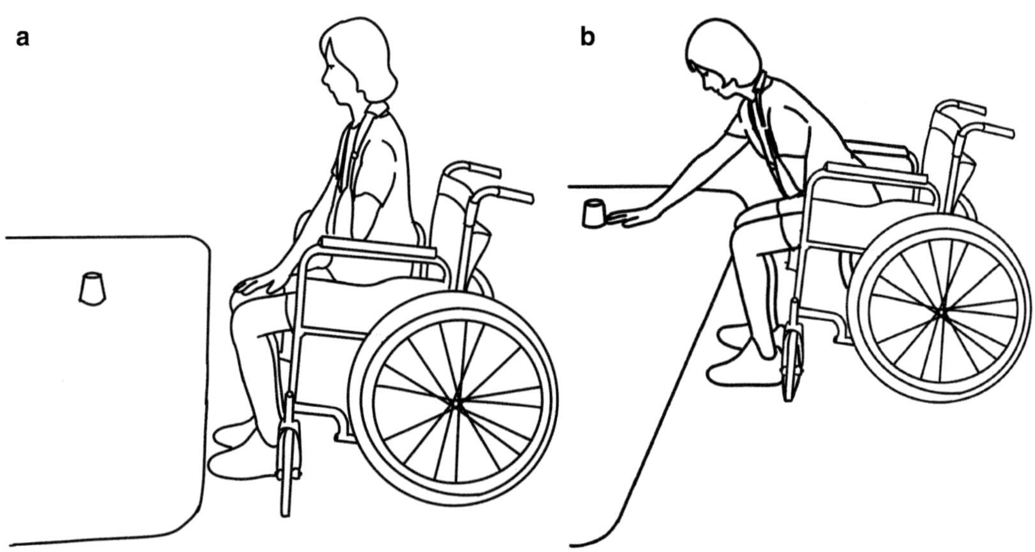

Fig. 10.4 Forward reaching training using a paper cup on a mat. Paper cup on the mat can help train more effectively by providing clear target. (**a**) Starting position, (**b**) Final position

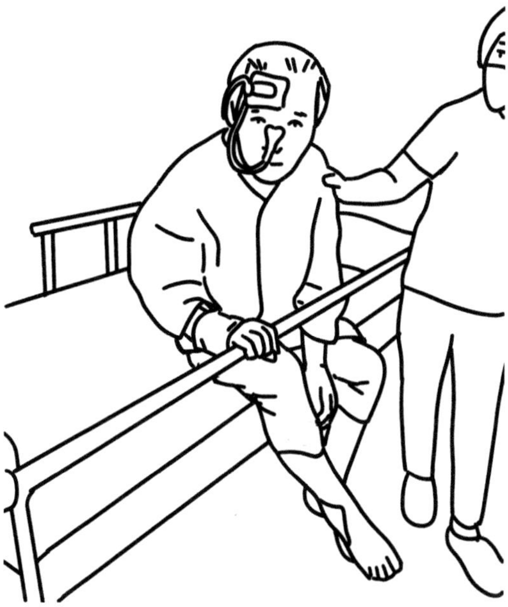

Fig. 10.5 Increasing safety by installing rods while performing sitting balance training

port using a pillow is not recommended due to the risk of learned nonuse. If a person has problems in both the sagittal and coronal planes simultaneously, it may be better to start training in the coronal plane first.

For individuals who have difficulty moving from the bed to a wheelchair, balance training can be performed while sitting on the edge of the bed. To ensure further safety, a rod can be set up at the side of the hospital bed (Fig. 10.5).

10.3.4 Reactive Balance Training

Reactive balance can be trained using unpredictable pushes. However, it is recommended that this only be implemented after proactive balance training has been regained.

10.4 Standing Balance Training

10.4.1 Steady-State Balance Training

10.4.1.1 Steady-State Balance Training with Both Lower Limbs

To maintain upright standing, sufficient muscle strength to support one's body weight is essential. If a patient has profound muscle weakness in the affected lower extremity, strengthening should be done before standing balance training commences.

Despite having sufficient muscle strength, some people may have difficulty standing without using their hands due to severe balance problems. In such cases, a therapeutic table and wall can be used.

Standing while placing both hands on the top of a table is easier for people with balance problems than standing with their hands rest on a wall. However, propping one's hands on the top of a therapeutic table can lead to learned nonuse of the affected lower limb. If possible, standing while touching the wall with a hand (or hands) is better than standing while propping one's hands on a table.

If people cannot maintain a standing position while using a therapeutic mat or when touching the wall, they may require the experience of forward movement of the center of mass using the forward reaching-in-a-sitting position or the sit-to-stand. Holding a bar and pulling the body forward is not recommended as it may encourage hand use and lead to learned nonuse of the lower extremity.

Some people with upper motor neuron lesions stand with abnormal postures, such as with no heel contact, hip and knee joint flexion, or genu recurvatum. If correction of these abnormal postures is impossible, it is necessary to delay training in a standing posture. Muscle strengthening and motor control training of the muscles in the affected lower limb may be helpful in correcting these problems.

Even when touching the wall with a hand, some people tilt and fall to the lateral side. If another wall (or corner of two walls) is nearby, people with a balance problem may tilt toward the wall without realizing it. If the wall is located in the opposite direction of a fall, the center of mass will move to the opposite direction of the fall, thus preventing it. Not only standing while keeping contact with the wall on the affected side, but also standing near the wall may be helpful in shifting the center of mass. Therefore, standing near the corner of a wall, keeping the falling side opposite the wall, may be helpful to maintain a standing posture.

If subjects can maintain a standing posture while touching a wall with their hands, the next step in training is the correction of asymmetric weight-bearing. The causes of weight-bearing asymmetry are diverse and may include motor weakness, asymmetric muscle tone, somatosensory deficits, neglect syndrome, distorted body schema, and impaired perception related to visual and postural vertical (Shumway-Cook et al. 2023). Weight-bearing asymmetry may also be a compensatory strategy in patients with significant motor impairment (de Haart et al. 2004). The direction of lateral tilt may face either the affected side or the unaffected side. Weakness of the affected side or impaired vertical sense is the main cause of a posture that has them tilting toward the affected side.

Correction of asymmetric weight-bearing can be achieved using several methods, such as education, motor control training, sensory feedback, nudging, changes in hand position on the wall, and mechanical disadvantage. Education is the first step in achieving symmetric standing. If people maintain a standing position with asymmetric weight-bearing, they need to be encouraged to bear weight more symmetrically. To regain normal gait, maximizing the function of the affected lower limb is absolutely necessary. The amount of weight-bearing on each lower extremity can be provided through proprioception (i.e., internal feedback) or external feedback, such as a body scale. Although it is possible to provide feedback to correct weight-bearing asymmetry using a body scale, a balance trainer, or a mirror, it is better for a subject to rely on their own somatosensory sense in order to stand symmetrically. If people cannot correct asymmetric standing, external sensory feedback may be helpful in achieving a symmetric standing posture. External feedback, such as visual feedback using a mirror, can be used. Alternatively, the position of the center of pressure can be monitored using a force plate.

By having people stand beside a wall, the center of mass can be moved to the less weight-bearing side. Not only standing with contact with the wall, but also standing near the wall may be helpful in shifting one's center of mass. Additionally, changing one's hand position on the wall may be helpful. By moving the hand position to the less weight-bearing side, the center of mass can be shifted to that side. It is also possible to place the unaffected lower limb at a mechanical disadvantage by placing the unaffected side on the top of a step. This mechanical disadvantage may be helpful in correcting an asymmetric standing posture.

Many people with gait disabilities maintain a standing position with their lower extremities in flexion. In this case, training to achieve standing with the lower extremities in extension is necessary. There are many strategies that can be used to correct a standing posture with the lower extremities in flexion, including stretching the joint contractures of the lower extremities, strengthening body weight support muscles, and practicing extension of the lower extremities in a standing posture.

Some people show unintentional forward rotation of the affected pelvis, which can be caused by weakness of the calf muscles. Testing and strengthening can be helpful in correcting this problem. Some people stand with excessive forward leaning against a wall. In such cases, asking people to bear more weight on the heel than on the forefoot may be helpful. To put more weight on the heel, people need to move their center of mass posteriorly, which leads to less use of the hands (Fig. 10.6).

By training with this method, people can lift their hands more easily.

With proper vertical alignment and symmetric weight-bearing, the pressure on the hands becomes minimal. Afterward, the subject can lift their hands from the wall and maintain an upright standing position.

If a patient can maintain a standing position without hand use, gradually increase the time of standing without hand use. Some patients have great difficulty maintaining a steady standing position for a long time and may lose their balance and fall. In such cases, setting a short target time can help the patient experience success and improve motivation.

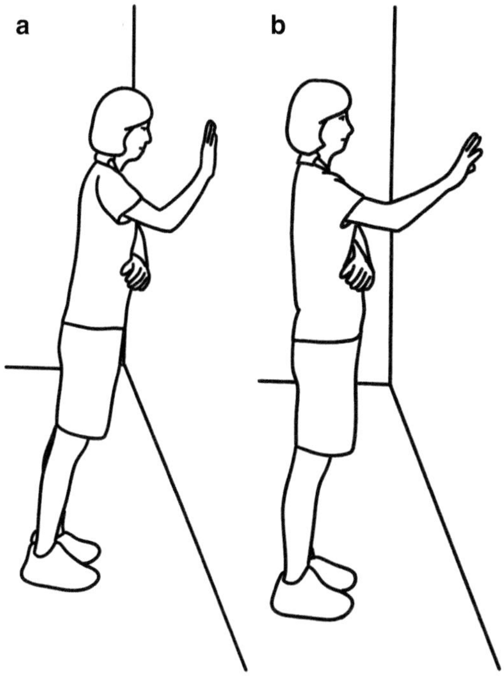

Fig. 10.6 Correction of forward leaning against a wall. Effective balance training is difficult to achieve when people lean body against the wall. Correction of forward leaning against a wall can be done by asking people to bear more weight on the heel than on the forefoot. (**a**) Forward learning against a wall, (**b**) Correction of forward leaning against a wall

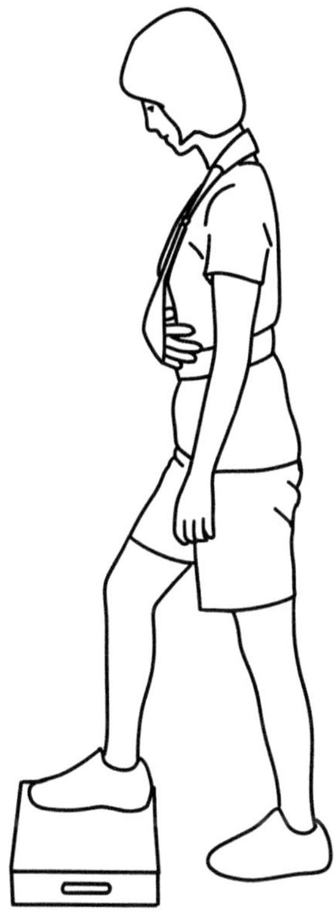

Fig. 10.7 Standing maintenance with foot on the top of a step

If the subject can maintain an upright symmetric standing position with their feet apart and without using their hands, training can move on to the next step. Standing can be made more difficult by placing one foot on the top of a step.

10.4.1.2 Steady-State Balance Training with a Step

Progression of training can be done by using a step, changing the position of the foot, or closing the eyes. It is more difficult to maintain a standing position with feet together, or with one foot in tandem. Standing can also be made more difficult by placing the affected foot on top of the step (Fig. 10.7).

A step with a height of 7.5 cm, a depth of 30 cm, and a width of 50 cm is widely used in clinical practice and research. The difficulty of training can be changed by altering the position of the feet. Increasing the distance between the feet increases the difficulty of the training. Maintaining a standing position with one foot on the step is more task-specific than other methods as it leads into the next step in training, which is stepping up.

Initially, instruct the subject to place the affected foot on the step with minimal weight-bearing and maintain an upright standing position. At the initial stage of training, touching the wall with one's hands may be helpful. If the person can maintain an upright standing position without using their hands and while displaying good performance (e.g., displaying minimal sway) for 1 min, training can progress by applying more weight-bearing on the foot placed on the step.

10.4.1.3 Single-Leg Standing

Single-leg standing can be used for steady-state balance training. Start by standing with both lower limbs and feet shoulder-width apart. Then lift the unaffected lower limb and maintain a single-leg standing position for as long as possible.

10.4.2 Proactive Balance Training

10.4.2.1 Weight Shift at Level Ground

The first step of dynamic balance training is weight shifting in a standing position. After the patient can maintain a standing position for more than 30 s without using their hands, it is possible to start weight-shift training in a standing posture near the wall.

Weight-shift training in a standing position can be done using various foot positions, such as standing with parallel feet, standing with diagonal foot positioning, or in a tandem stance. Weight shifting in a standing position with diagonal foot positioning is very useful for balance training and task-oriented training. To accomplish this, have the subject place the affected limb anterior to the unaffected limb and gradually increase the weight-bearing on affected the lower limbs.

In this training, the degree of weight shift is a critical component, and the amount of weight shift can be assessed using somatosensory senses or a body weight scale. Although a body weight scale is effective for providing information about the amount of weight shift, patients must flex their head to see the scale, which is not desirable. Rather, it is better to provide information at eye level, allowing patients to see the information while maintaining an upright standing posture. With enough weight shift, the heel of the unaffected foot may lift automatically. However, if the heel does not lift automatically, voluntary heel lifting of the unaffected foot may be helpful in shifting the weight to the affected lower limb. After the patient regains the ability to shift their weight fully to the affected limb, they can briefly lift the affected limb.

10.4.2.2 Weight Shift with a Step

Proactive balance can be trained using weight shifting in a standing position with the affected foot on top of a step. This is considered task-oriented training as after mastering weight shift training, step-up training follows.

To begin, instruct the subject to stand close to the wall, facing it while on both legs. Next, have them place the affected foot on the step, which is to be positioned between the wall and the subject. They may touch the wall with their hands if necessary. While maintaining a standing balance, the subject should shift their weight to the affected lower limb as much as possible. Then they need to shift their weight to the unaffected lower limb and take a brief rest. Repeat this sequence as necessary (Fig. 10.8).

With improvement in balance, the use of hands should be minimized, utilizing only light touch or no hand usage at all. During this training, maintaining knee flexion and vertical trunk alignment is important. To shift weight properly, the knee joint should be moved forward. Instructions such as "shift your knee above your big toe" may be helpful for individuals to understand the kinematics of the task.

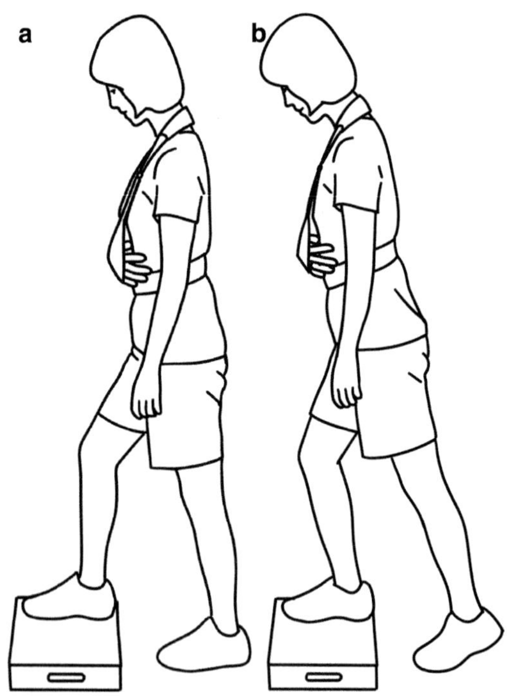

Fig. 10.8 Weight shift with a step. If it is impossible or dangerous to perform the step-up, balance ability can be improved by performing weight shift to the affected lower extremity with the affected foot on the top of the step. (**a**) Starting position, (**b**) Final position

Additionally, providing variable training is important in order to make it possible to use the trained task in the real world. However, using many steps with different heights in training can be challenging. Variable training can still be achieved with only one kind of step by changing the foot's location. Increasing the distance between the feet requires more flexion of the joints of the stance limb and causes the task to be more difficult.

10.4.2.3 Step-Up

For healthy individuals, going downstairs is easier than going upstairs, but going downstairs is more challenging for people with balance problems, osteoarthritis, and paresis due to upper motor neuron lesions. Step-up is the second step of dynamic balance training.

During step-up training, it is recommended that the subject stands close to the wall and faces the wall. In the initial stages of step-up training, touching the wall with their hands is acceptable. However, as training progresses, hand usage should be minimized and eventually stopped. To minimize pressure on the hands, standing upright is essential. Even if people do not touch the wall with their hands, the wall can help prevent falling when balance is lost, thus alleviating the fear of falling.

The step-up exercise can be divided into ascending and descending phases. It may be necessary to touch the wall with the hand during the descending phase because it is more difficult and potentially more dangerous than the ascending phase.

Step-up training can further be divided into lateral step-up and forward step-up. Because lateral step-up is easier than forward step-up, lateral step-up can be trained before progressing to forward step-up training. To perform a lateral step-up, follow these steps: Begin by standing on both legs near the wall, facing the wall, with the step on the affected side. Place the affected foot on the distant part of the top of the step while the unaffected foot remains on the floor. Shift body weight to the affected limb and lift the unaffected limb, placing it on the step (Fig. 10.9).

Returning the unaffected foot to the floor is more challenging because it requires eccentric contraction of the affected limb. Touching the wall can be used during the return to the starting position.

The forward step-up is performed as follows: Begin by placing the step near the wall and standing on both legs close to the step, facing the wall. Then place the affected foot on the top of the step. Shift body weight to the affected foot and lift the unaffected foot, placing it on the top of the step (Fig. 10.10).

To shift weight properly during the step-up, it is important to move the knee joint forward. Therefore, the following instructions can be helpful. Start by moving the knee joint above the big toe of the affected foot, and then shift body weight to the affected foot. Next, lift the unaffected lower limb and softly place it on the step.

Returning to the starting position during the step-up can be more challenging than the actual step-up. Touching the wall can be used during the return to the starting position if needed.

If a patient can perform the step-up movement while demonstrating good performance and without using their hands, the training can progress to the next step, which is the step-down.

Some patients may exhibit near-buckling or genu recurvatum during the step-up movement. Since this abnormal movement can become a habitual pattern and interfere the recovery of normal gait, it is important to prevent it. Educating the patient about the importance of preventing abnormal movements can be helpful. If preventing these abnormal movements is impossible, step-up training should be delayed. In such cases, training can be done with a partial step-up.

A partial step-up starts in the same position as the forward step-up. After shifting the weight to the affected lower limb, briefly lift the entire unaffected foot and return to the initial position. Maintain knee flexion during this training. If the patient can briefly lift the unaffected foot while maintaining balance for several seconds, training can progress to the full step-up.

It is crucial to perform the step-up with slow, smooth, and controlled movements. Performing a

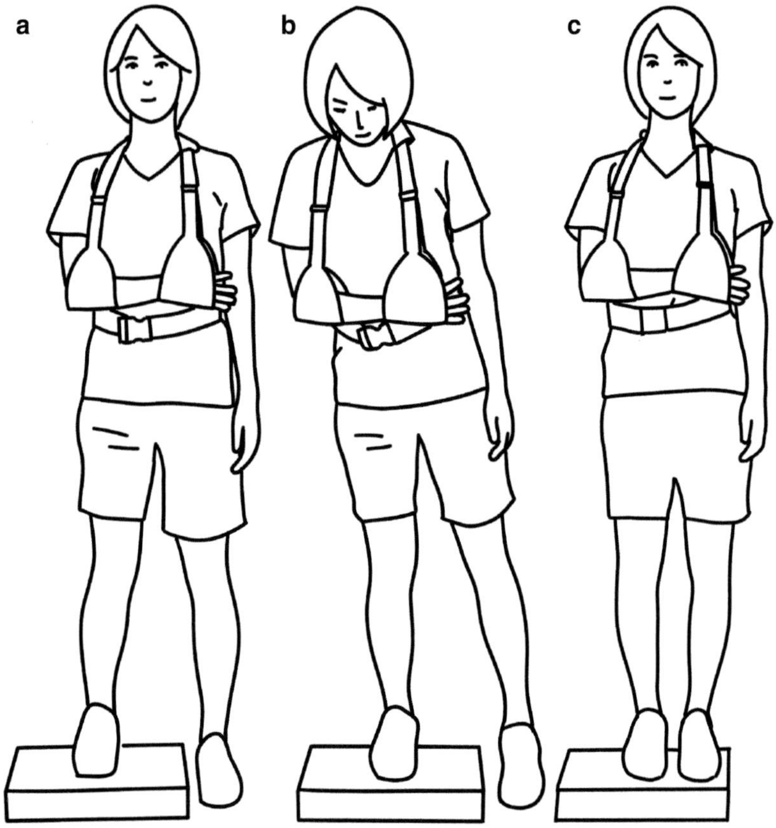

Fig. 10.9 Lateral step-up movement. It is easier to do lateral step-up than to do forward step-up. If the progress of the balance training is slow, the balance training can be performed by lateral step-up. (**a**) Starting position, (**b**) Midpoint of lateral step-up, (**c**) Final position

step-up with hand support on a table is not recommended as it can lead to the undue use of the hand to support body weight, potentially causing learned nonuse of the affected lower limb.

Some patients may have difficulty maintaining tibia alignment vertically in the coronal plane during step-up. This abnormal alignment can lead to poor performance and an increased risk of injury. Education and strengthening exercises for the hip internal rotators may be helpful in correcting this poor alignment.

10.4.2.4 Step-Down Movement

For step-down training, start by placing a step near the wall with enough space to allow for stepping down. Stand on top of the step with both lower limbs while facing the wall. Lift the unaffected foot and descend to the floor. Then lift the unaffected foot and return to the starting position (Fig. 10.11).

In the initial stages of training, touching the wall can aid in maintaining balance. As training progresses, hand usage should gradually decrease and eventually stop.

Performing a slow and controlled step-down is more challenging than performing a rapid one. It is important to execute the step-down with a smooth and controlled movement. Keeping a mental image of a paper cup on top of the head or actually balancing a paper cup on the head can help in achieving controlled movement.

10.4.2.5 Step-Down-Touch (-the-Floor)

A step-down-touch is similar to a step-down movement performed extremely slowly. To conduct step-down-touch training, position a step near the wall with adequate space for stepping down and touching the floor. Stand on top of the step with both lower limbs while facing the wall. Lift the unaffected foot and gently touch the floor. Then lift the unaffected foot and return to the starting position (Fig. 10.12).

During the initial stage of training, touching the wall can be helpful for maintaining balance

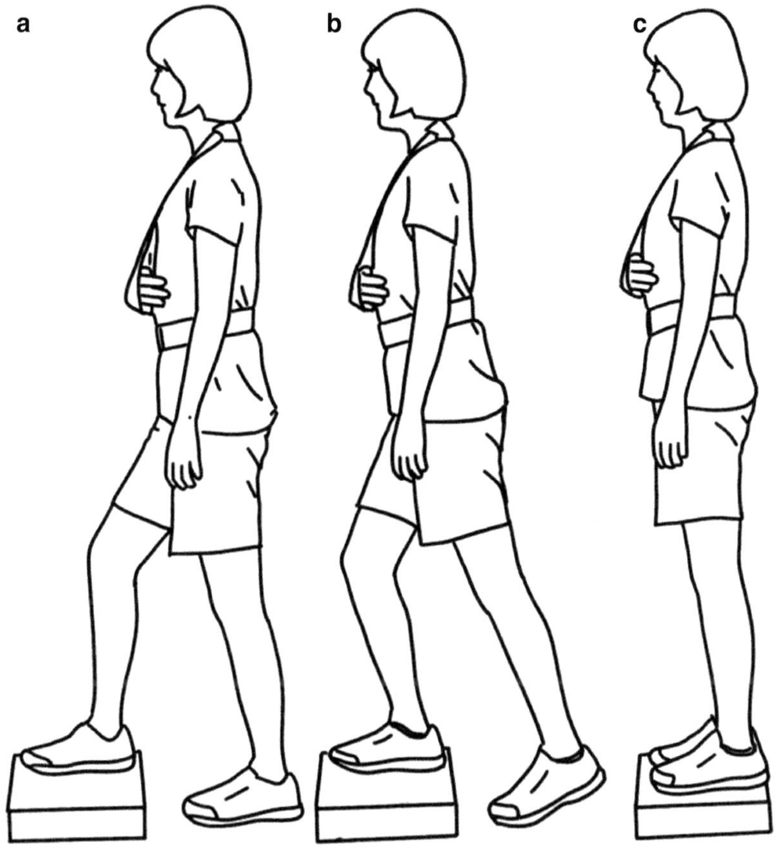

Fig. 10.10 Forward step-up. Balance ability can be improved by placing the affected foot on the top of the step and slowly lifting the entire body over the step. (**a**) Starting position, (**b**) Midpoint of forward step-up, (**c**) Final position

during step-down-touch exercises. However, with continued training, hand usage should gradually decrease and eventually stop. Touching can be done with the forefoot, the whole foot, or the heel. Touching the floor with the heel is the most challenging variant. If individuals lack strength in the ankle plantar flexors, performing step-down-touch is impossible. Therefore, it is essential to regain strength in the ankle plantar flexors before starting this training. Providing instructions such as "imagine touching a pin gently with your heel" can aid in performing step-down-touch exercises more softly.

Step-down-touch training offers several advantages. First, it provides a clear target, which is the floor, and marking the floor can make the target even clearer. This exercise also does not require expensive equipment and manages to closely mimic the movement of the supporting lower limb during gait.

However, it is crucial to note that there is a risk of falling during training with the step-down-touch. Therefore, supervision by another person or the use of an overhead harness may be necessary to prevent falls.

10.4.2.6 Single-Leg (Mini) Squat

Although the single-leg squat is commonly utilized in sports rehabilitation to assess strength and balance, it can also be incorporated into balance training. The single-leg squat and step-down exercises share a similar movement pattern during the descent phase at the hip and knee joints (Lewis et al. 2015).

To perform a single-leg squat, stand on both legs close to the wall, facing the wall. Then lift the unaffected foot and keep it lifted. Flex the affected lower limb while maintaining standing balance. For safety, placing a chair behind the individual may be helpful (Fig. 10.13).

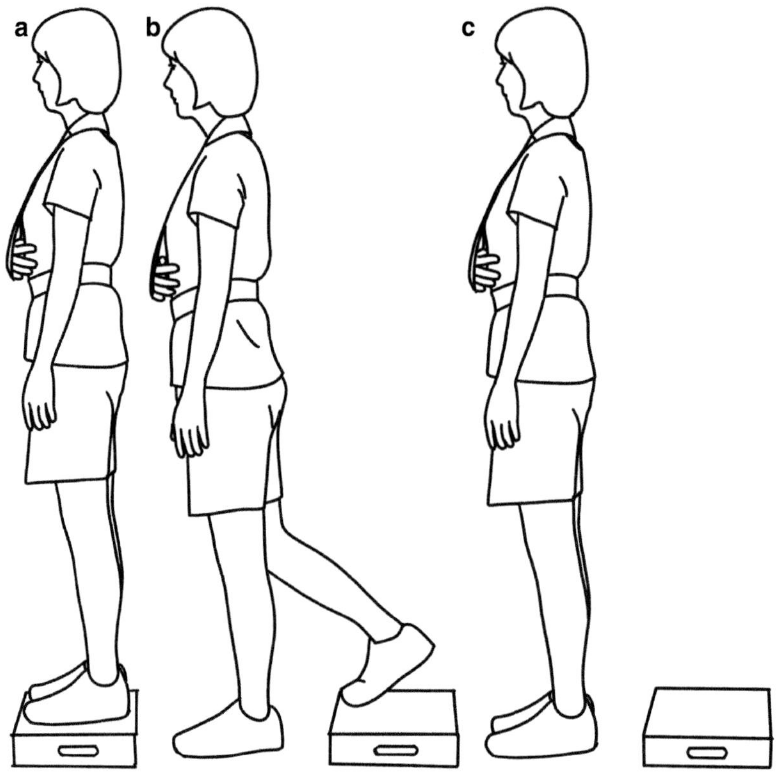

Fig. 10.11 Step-down. Stand on the step and place the floor with unaffected foot. (**a**) Starting position, (**b**) Midpoint of step-down, (**c**) Final position

When using the single-leg squat for balance training, the most crucial aspect is executing the single-leg squat with slow, smooth, and controlled movements. Imagining a paper cup on top of the head or actually placing one there can help promote controlled movement.

If individuals with balance problems can perform the single-leg squat with a small range of motion while maintaining standing balance, they can gradually increase the range of motion to progress their training. To enhance dynamic balance training, minimizing the use of hand support is essential. Performing the single-leg squat with more weight-bearing on the heel than the forefoot helps maintain an extended posture and prevents leaning forward.

However, it is impossible to perform a single-leg squat without adequate strength in the ankle plantar flexors. Therefore, individuals should focus on regaining strength in the ankle plantar flexors before starting single-leg squat training.

The single-leg squat offers many advantages. First, it does not require any equipment and is relatively safe. The horizontal movement of the body during a single-leg squat is also minimal. Additionally, if the exercise is done between a wall and a bed, the risk of falling can be minimized, making it a useful approach for individuals who exercise alone at home. The placement of a large doll next to the individual can also serve to enhance safety even further.

One limitation of the single-leg squat is the absence of a clear target. While individuals with good cognition and sensory function can rely on their proprioception, those with balance problems may have difficulty perceiving the amount of flexion necessary during single-leg squat training. Providing external feedback to individuals regarding the amount of flexion in the weight-bearing lower extremity may be helpful. Ground reaction force changes with the vertical movement of the center of mass. By using vertical ground reaction force, the movement of the center of mass can also be indirectly evaluated. Electronic body weight scales or pressure sensors can be used to provide external feedback on body center of mass movement. To maintain an upright posture, the display should be at eye level.

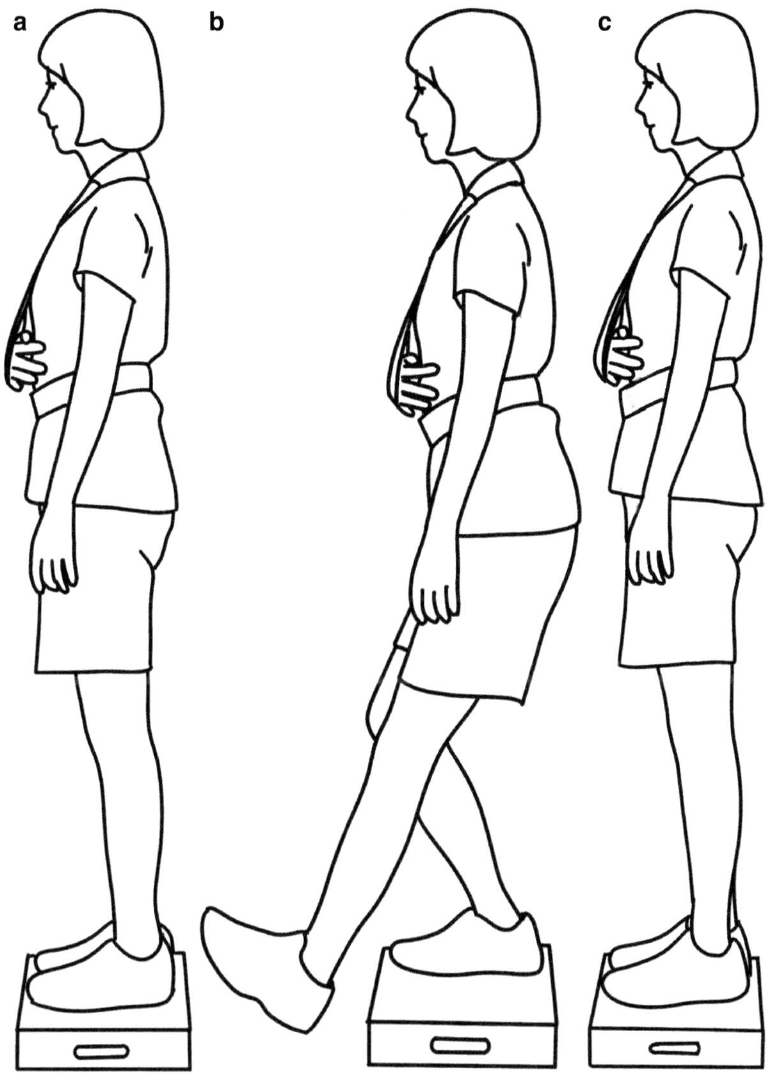

Fig. 10.12 Step-down-touch. Stand on the step and lightly touch the floor with the unaffected foot while supporting the entire weight with the affected foot. The heel of the affected foot remains in contact with the step. (**a**) Starting position, (**b**) Midpoint of step-down-touch, (**c**) Final position

10.4.2.7 Foot Reach

The foot-reach movement is a widely used exercise to train dynamic balance in various rehabilitation settings. To perform foot-reach training, stand on both legs close to the wall, leaving enough space for to perform the foot-reaching movement while facing the wall. Lift the unaffected foot, touch a target on the floor, and return to the starting position while maintaining standing balance. Markings on the floor can serve as target points for foot-reach exercises. By increasing the distance between the affected foot and the marking, the training can be progressively intensified. Foot-reach exercises can be performed in various directions, such as forward, backward, lateral, ipsilateral diagonal, and opposite diagonal (braiding) (Fig. 10.14). It is important to maintain heel contact to the floor when doing foot-reach training.

It is important to perform the foot-reach with slow, smooth, and controlled movements. Imagining a paper cup on top of the head or actually placing one there can be helpful for promoting controlled movements.

The foot-reach offers several advantages. For example, it involves a clear target when markings are used on the floor, does not require any equipment, and closely resembles the movement of the

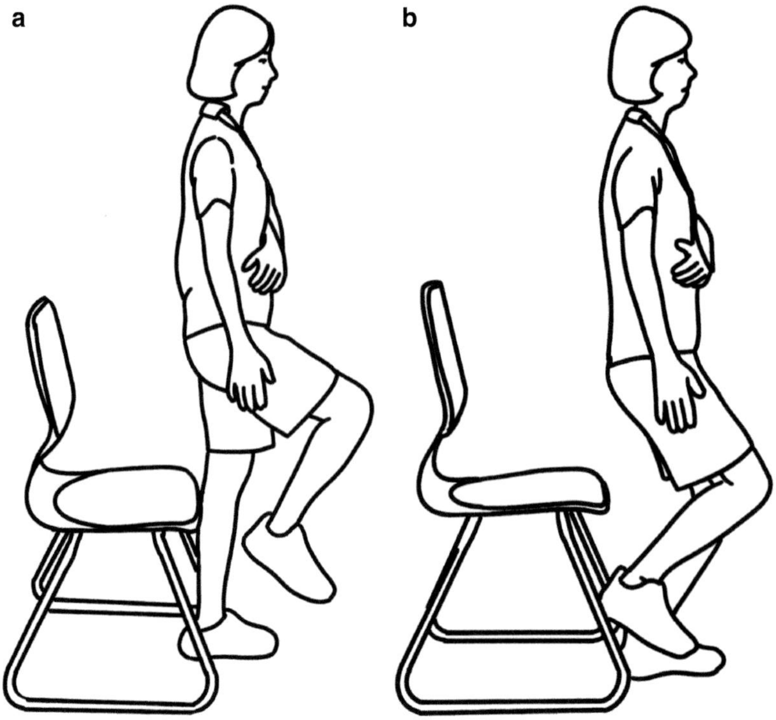

Fig. 10.13 Single-leg squat. Stand on the affected lower extremity and flex and extend the lower extremity to the extent that it can be controlled. The chair immediately behind people can contribute to protecting the body when falling. (**a**) Starting position, (**b**) Final position

lower limbs in stance period during the gait cycle. However, there is a risk of falling during foot-reach training, so it may be necessary to have someone else present to provide assistance. Otherwise, consider using an overhead harness for fall prevention.

10.4.2.8 Step Touch

The step-touch can also be utilized to train dynamic balance. To perform balance training with the step-touch, place the step near the wall and stand on both legs close to the step, facing the wall. Then lift the unaffected foot and touch the top of the step before returning to the starting position. Repeat this movement, and the affected foot can also be used to touch the top of the step (Fig. 10.15).

During this task, the support of body weight is provided primarily by the extension state of a lower limb, which can make it easier than the step-up exercise. The step-touch can be useful for training the swing phase movement of the lower limb and can also help correct toe drag during gait.

During the initial stages of step-touch training, touching the wall with the hand can be used for support. However, as training progresses, it is essential to minimize hand usage, eventually performing step-touch without relying on hand use. Additionally, it is possible to increase the difficulty of step-touch training by using a higher step or by increasing the speed of the step-touch.

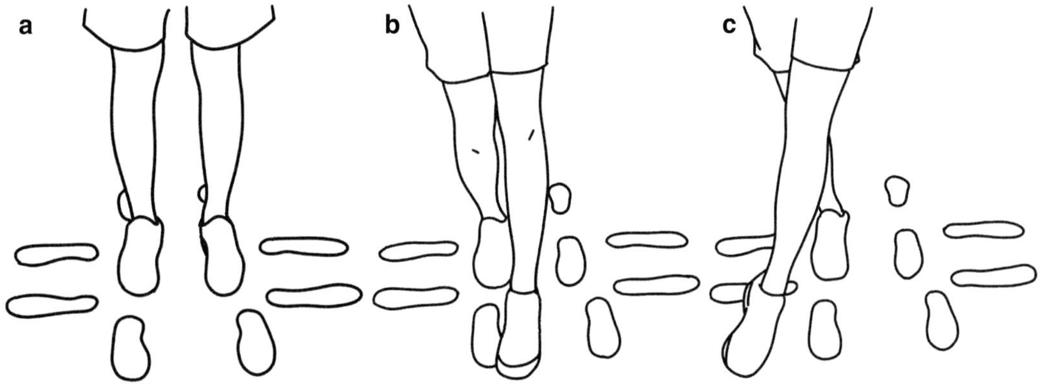

Fig. 10.14 Foot reach: (**a**) starting position; (**b**) foot reach forward; (**c**) foot reach opposite diagonal

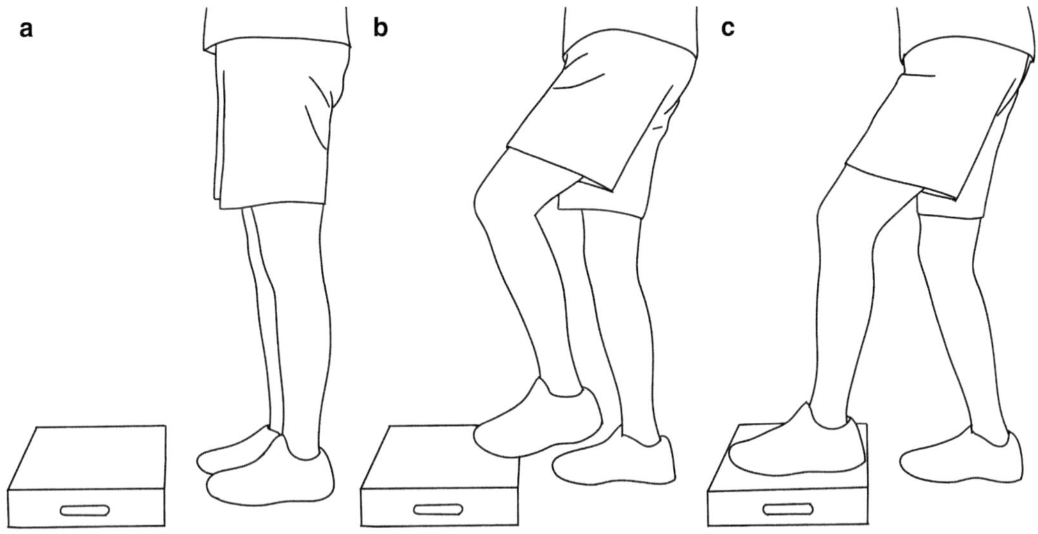

Fig. 10.15 Step-touch. Stand in front of the step and raise and lower the foot of the affected lower extremity on the top of the step. The main purpose of this training is the foot advancement of the affected lower extremity. (**a**) Starting position, (**b**) Midpoint of step-touch, (**c**) Final position

10.5 Balance Training with Equipment

Many clinical studies have evaluated the effectiveness of balance training using equipment, but its effectiveness has not been definitively established. Some balance trainers only provide information about horizontal movement of the center of mass, which may explain the mixed results seen in studies. However, there are balance trainers that incorporate both horizontal and vertical movement of the center of mass. These machines use strain gauges to measure lateral movement of the center of mass and tilting sensors on the thigh to measure lower limb flexion (Fig. 10.16).

Training with such equipment may be more effective for improving proactive balance.

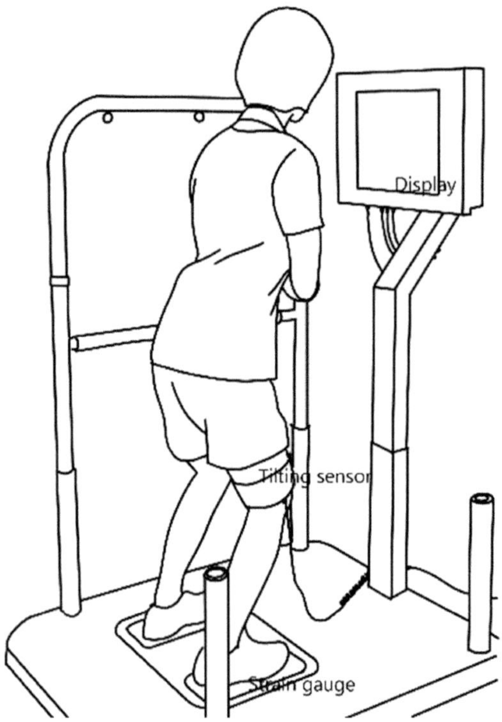

Fig. 10.16 Balance trainer that uses horizontal and vertical movement of the center of mass

10.6 Reactive Balance Training

Reactive balance training is essential for improving the ability to protect the body from falling, but it should be initiated only after dynamic balance has been regained.

Reactive balance to external purturbation can be divided into two strategies: in place stategy and change in support strategy.

External perturbation can be given by pushing the sternum, pulling the shoulder or pelvis and lean and release. Using moderate external perturbation, it is possible to train to restore balance using in place strategy, without moving the feet and without use hands. With large external perturbation, it is possible to train reactive balance using change in support strategy, take a step or reach hand for support.

During reactive balance training, it is crucial that people be protected from falling. Using an overhead harness is an effective strategy for fall prevention.

10.7 Summary

The difficulty of the task can be increased by reducing the base of support and sensory input, increasing the magnitude of movement, increasing the requirement for precise control of movement, and introducing dual tasks.

To make balance training effective, it is essential that the area of the base of support be minimized and that hand usage be reduced in order to improve balance. Using the hands to support balance extends the base of support and may lead to learned nonuse of the affected lower limb, potentially interfering with the recovery of normal gait. Therefore, hand usage should be minimized for effective balance training.

To improve proactive balance, it is necessary to move the center of mass not only horizontally but also vertically.

Dynamic sitting balance training can be done by reaching forward and then returning to the starting position while the hands are on top of a table, bed, or lapboard. With the improvement of sitting balance, this movement can be done with the subject's hands in the air.

For healthy individuals, going downstairs is easier than going upstairs, but going downstairs is more challenging for people with balance problems, osteoarthritis, and paresis due to the presence of upper motor neuron lesions.

If individuals lack strength in the ankle plantar flexors, performing step-down-touch-the-floor exercises may be impossible. Therefore, it is essential to regain strength in the ankle plantar flexors before starting this training.

References

Allen NE, Sherrington C, Paul SS, Canning CG. Balance and falls in Parkinson's disease: a meta-analysis of the effect of exercise and motor training. Mov Disord. 2011;26(9):1605–15.

American College of Sports Medicine, Chodzko-Zajko WJ, Proctor DN, Singh MAF, Minson CT, Nigg CR, Salem GJ, Skinner JS. American College of Sports Medicine position stand. Exercise and physical activity for older adults. Med Sci Sports Exerc. 2009;41(7):1510–30.

de Haart M, Geurts AC, Huidekoper SC, Fasotti L, van Limbeek J. Recovery of standing balance in postacute stroke patients: a rehabilitation cohort study. Arch Phys Med Rehabil. 2004;85(6):886–95.

Lesinski M, Hortobágyi T, Muehlbauer T, Gollhofer A, Granacher U. Effects of balance training on balance performance in healthy older adults: a systematic review and meta-analysis. Sports Med. 2015;45:1721–38.

Lewis CL, Foch E, Luko MM, Loverro KL, Khuu A. Differences in lower extremity and trunk kinematics between single leg squat and step down tasks. PLoS One. 2015;10(5):e0126258.

Sherrington C, Tiedemann A, Fairhall N, Close JCT, Lord SR. Exercise to prevent falls in older adults: an updated meta-analysis and best practice recommendations. N S W Public Health Bull. 2011;22(3–4):78–83.

Shumway-Cook A, Woollacott MH, Rachwani J, Santamaria V. Abnormal postural control (Chapter 10). In: Motor control: translating research into clinical practice. 6th ed. Philadelphia: Lippincott Williams & Wilkins; 2023. p. 247–80.

11 Flexibility

11.1 Importance of Flexibility

Flexibility is essential to normal gait. Loss of flexibility is caused by neural and non-neural causes, which can lead to abnormal gait, increased energy cost, and an increased risk of falling.

11.2 Maintaining Flexibility

Flexibility can be maintained through the active range of motion exercise or by the passive range of motion and positioning of body segments in a stretched position. Maintaining flexibility and preventing the loss of flexibility are the best strategies. If there is a loss of flexibility, restoration of flexibility is absolutely necessary. Stretching can be accomplished via manual stretching, serial casting, orthosis, or with the help of machines.

11.3 Principles of Stretching

11.3.1 Focused Stretching

Stretching must be focused on the target structure. If a stretching force is spread out to other structures, it may cause more harm than good. For example, when stretching the ankle joint, decreasing the angle of toe out is very important. Eversion of the subtalar joint can cause the intertarsal joints (e.g., naviculocuboidal joint and caneocuboidal joint) to become more mobile. In that state, an external force stretch not only the ankle joint but also the intertrarsal joints. By decreasing the angle of toe out, the subtalar joint is inverted, which causes the external force to act more selectively in stretching out the ankle joint (Perry and Burnfield 2010).

11.3.2 Minimize Resistance to Stretching

Muscle tone changes according to posture. Due to postural tone, muscle tone is low in a lying-down posture and high in a standing posture. Therefore, stretching in a lying-down position is superior to stretching in a standing position.

Discomfort or pain may cause muscle contraction and interfere with proper stretching. Therefore, discomfort when stretching must be minimized. To minimize discomfort, it should be done in a slow and gentle manner.

Rapid stretching may induce reflective contraction of muscles, thus leading to tissue damage.

11.3.3 Appropriate Amount of Stretching

To be effective and safe, stretching should be done with appropriate force. If the amount of stretching is inadequate, it may be ineffective.

Y.-S. Lee, *Task Oriented Gait Training*, https://doi.org/10.1007/978-981-97-3348-4_11

However, if the amount of stretching is excessive, it may cause pain, tissue damage, and may even result in aggravated contracture.

The amount of stretching can be divided by the resistance to stretching. At the initial stage of stretching, the slack in the connective tissue is removed, so there is no change of resistance or only a minimal change of resistance. This can be considered the horizontal region as there is no increase in resistance due to stretching.

The next stage is the transitional region, which is located between the horizontal region and the exponential region. In this region, resistance increases gradually with further stretching.

The final stage is the exponential region. In this stage, resistance to stretching is increased exponentially, nearly reaching a vertical (Hunter and Brown 2009).

Stretching in the middle of the transitional region may be considered the optimal region of stretching (Fig. 11.1).

11.3.4 Sustained Stretch

To be an effective stretch, maintaining the stretched position for as long as possible is necessary (Light et al. 1984). To perform sustained stretching, many methods are used, such as manual stretching, orthoses, serial casting, or the use of a tilt table or sliding tilt table.

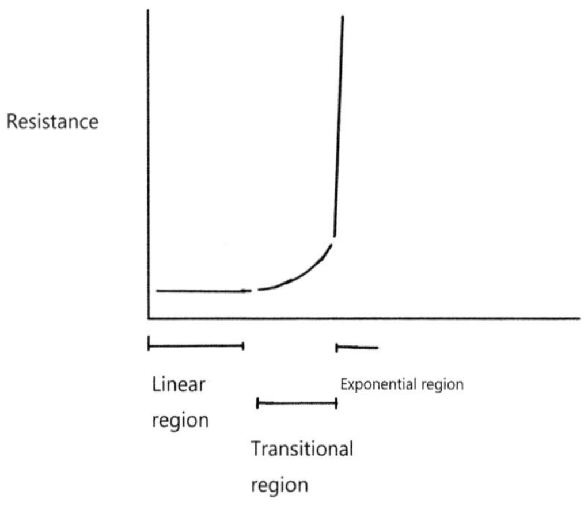

Fig. 11.1 Relation between stretching and resistance

11.4 Methods of Stretching

11.4.1 Manual Stretching

Manual stretching is used most commonly to stretch tissue contracture. It is effective at restoring flexibility, does not need special equipment, and can apply to any body structure. Therefore, it is often the first method used.

If stretching is conducted appropriately, the risk of adverse effects is very low.

However, manual stretching has several limitations. Since it requires the use of manpower, it may come at a relatively high cost. In addition, it is difficult to perform sustained stretching simply through manual stretching. Finally, it is difficult to stretch rigid contractures or contractures of the ankle joint as the calf muscles are large while the lever arm of the foot is short (Perry and Burnfield 2010).

11.4.2 Stretching with Orthosis

Maintaining a stretched position (i.e., sustained stretching) is an essential component of effective stretching. For sustained stretching, orthoses can be used. However, the use of orthoses for the purpose of stretching may require a customized orthosis, which is often quite expensive and may cause inconvenience and discomfort for people with a contracture.

11.4.3 Serial Casting

Serial casting can be used to perform sustained stretching. Although it is effective at stretching a body structure with a contracture, it causes discomfort and may even cause severe complications, such as skin necrosis. Therefore, it is not commonly used.

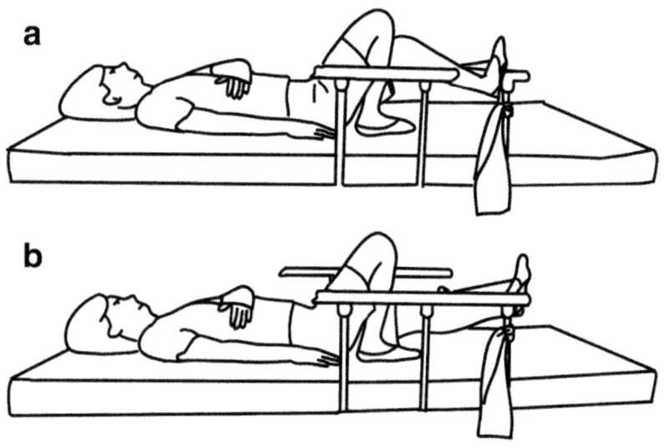

Fig. 11.2 Active motion of the knee joint with an elastic band. The elasticity of the rubber band fixed to the safety bars can help flex the knee joint. (**a**) Knee flexion, (**b**) Knee extension

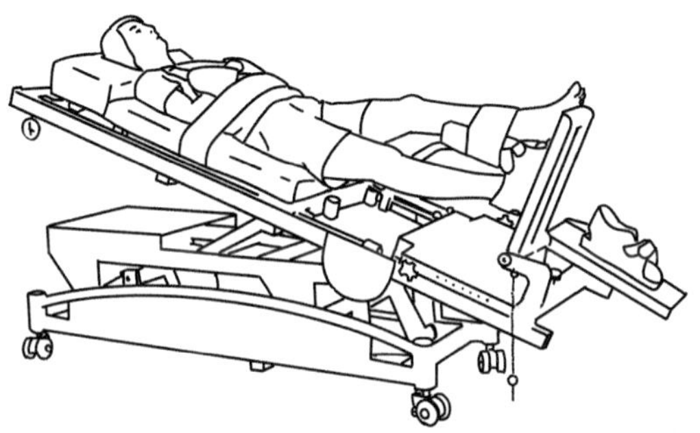

Fig. 11.3 Ankle stretching using a sliding tilt table

11.4.4 Stretching in a Standing Posture

Although weight bearing in a standing posture can be used to perform stretching of the ankle joint, it is very difficult for people with severe motor weakness or balance problems. Additionally, it is difficult to adjust the stretching force in this position. Therefore, stretching with tilt table or sliding tilt table may be more useful.

11.4.5 Stretching with a Machine

11.4.5.1 Continuous Passive Motion Machine

A continuous passive motion machine is very useful for making passive motion of the knee joint, especially after surgery. If people can move more actively, active motion of the knee joint may be more beneficial than passive motion caused by a continuous passive motion machine. In addition, active motion can be assisted with the use of a rubber band (Fig. 11.2).

11.4.5.2 Tilt Table

Using a tilt table allows for easy stretching of the ankle plantar flexor. Since stretching is done in a lying-down position, the muscle is relaxed during stretching. Additionally, the stretching force can be changed easily by changing the tilting angle.

Due to friction between the subject and the sliding top, the angle of the tilt table is larger than the angle of a sliding tilt table for the purpose of stretching. Thus, it may cause excessive force and discomfort of the ankle joint. This may decrease the effectiveness of the stretching.

11.4.5.3 Sliding Tilt Table

When stretching the ankle joint with a sliding tilt table, the body and the sliding top move together, so there is minimized friction between the sliding top and tilting frame (Fig. 11.3).

The angle of the sliding tilt table, which causes the sliding table to move downward, is quite small. Stretching with a sliding tilt table may be more comfortable for people than stretching with a tilt table because the smaller inclination angle can be used to more easily facilitate stretching due to the decreased friction of the downward movement. Additionally, it can minimize discomfort, facilitate muscle relaxation, and may even maximize the effectiveness of the stretching.

The angle of the foot plate is important for effective stretching. If the heel is not in contact with the footplate due to ankle contracture, stretching may cause discomfort and may even decrease the effectiveness of the stretching.

The optimal angle of the foot plate is an angle at which the heel contact foot plate reaches in a short time after initiation of the stretching and which does not cause pain. If the heel does not contact the foot plate, people may feel pain, so it would be very difficult to relax the calf muscles. Toe down rotation of the foot plate can solve this problem.

11.5 Summary

For effective stretching, it is necessary to use the appropriate amount of stretching and prolonged stretching.

The amount of stretching can be divided by the resistances to stretching: the horizontal region, the transitional region, and the vertical region. In the transitional region, resistance is increased gradually with further stretching. Stretching in the middle of the transitional region may be the optimal region of stretching.

To perform sustained stretching, many methods are utilized, such as orthoses, serial casting, a tilt table, or a sliding tilt table.

Stretching with a sliding tilt table may be more comfortable for people than stretching with a tilt table because the smaller inclination angle can be used to stretch due to the reduced friction caused in the downward movement. In addition, it can minimize discomfort, facilitate muscle relaxation, and may even maximize the effectiveness of the stretching.

References

Hunter SK, Brown DA. Muscle: the primary stabilizer and mover of the skeletal system. In: Neumann DA, editor. Kinesiology of the musculoskeletal system: foundations for rehabilitation. 2nd ed. St. Louis: Mosby; 2009. p. 47–76.

Light KE, Nuzik S, Personius W, Barstrom A. Low-load prolonged stretch vs. high-load brief stretch in treating knee contractures. Phys Ther. 1984;64(3):330–3.

Perry J, Burnfield J. Ankle foot complex. In: Gait analysis: normal and pathological function. 2nd ed. New Jersey: Slack Incorporated; 2010. p. 165–74.

Task-Specific Gait Training 12

12.1 Definition of Task-Specific Gait Training

Task-specific training follows the tenet that "gait is improved by the experience of gait." Sometimes this term is used interchangeably with task-oriented training; however, its scope is narrower than task-oriented training. In a more specific sense, it refers to training that uses gait itself to improve gait. For training individuals with severe impairments, external supports may be required, such as robots, body weight support systems, and assistance from other healthcare providers. It may also require expensive equipment and place a physical burden on people with gait disabilities and healthcare providers.

12.2 Level Ground (Overground) Gait Training

Gait training on level ground is the primary method of gait training. For people with mild impairments, training is done on level ground through diverse mobility tasks, such as walking forward, walking backward, walking sideways, stepping over obstacles, stepping around obstacles, and tandem gait. However, for people with severe impairments, massive external support is needed.

12.3 Gait Training with a Cane

The use of a cane increases the base of support and enhances standing balance. However, it may increase weight-bearing asymmetry between the two legs and lead to learned nonuse of the affected lower limb (Shumway-Cook et al. 2023).

12.4 Gait Training with Parallel Bars

Since parallel bars provide a stable base of support, people with gait disabilities use them to support their body weight. However, they may lead to learned nonuse of the affected lower limb. To reduce the usage of the upper extremities, sliding handles have been developed, increasing lower limb muscle activation and decreasing weight-bearing through the upper limbs (Stephenson et al. 2009).

12.5 Gait Training with a Treadmill

In gait training with a treadmill, people with gait disabilities have to match the speed of the treadmill, making it more challenging for them than simply walking on level ground. In many cases, people use

Y.-S. Lee, *Task Oriented Gait Training*, https://doi.org/10.1007/978-981-97-3348-4_12

handrails for safety, but this problem can be solved using an overhead harness. Training with a treadmill can increase gait speed and has several advantages: it does not require a large space, it is easier to use an overhead harness than with gait training on level ground, and passive extension of the hip joint may facilitate the activation of the hip flexors. However, it also has its limitations; it requires equipment and space, is less portable, and walking on a treadmill is different from walking on level ground, which may explain why the effectiveness of treadmill training is not always better than other gait training methods (Helbostad 2003).

12.6 Body Weight-Supported Training

12.6.1 Body Weight-Supported Overground Training

Body weight support makes walking possible for people with severe motor impairments. However, body weight-supported overground gait training has several limitations. First, it requires equipment and a large space. It is also more challenging to use a body weight support system compared to gait training on a treadmill. If the amount of body weight support is significant, it may cause discomfort and skin problems for people with gait disabilities.

12.6.2 Body Weight-Supported Treadmill Training

Body weight-supported treadmill training enables individuals who are unable to walk, even with assistance from walking aids or other forms of aid, to regain the ability to walk. It also allows for a higher dosage of training for those with limited walking function (Helbostad 2003). However, manual assistance is required for those with severe motor impairments, which may place a physical burden on healthcare providers. Furthermore, body weight-supported treadmill training has not shown superiority over conventional training in people recovering from a stroke (Duncan et al. 2011).

12.7 Gait Training with Functional Electrical Stimulation

Functional electrical stimulation can be employed to improve gait function. In a systematic review, it was found to enhance walking distance when evaluated using the 6-min walk test in chronic stroke patients. However, its effectiveness compared to other gait training approaches remains unclear (Pereira et al. 2012).

12.8 Gait Training with Robots

Robots enable task-specific gait training for individuals with severe motor impairments and can increase the amount of training they receive. Robots used on treadmills can be classified into exoskeleton types and end-effector types. Gait training with robots is already employed in many hospitals worldwide. However, gait training with robots faces several limitations. First of all, robots are highly expensive, making it challenging for many hospitals to afford them. Moreover, their superiority over other gait training methods remains unclear (Nedergård et al. 2021; Calafiore et al. 2022).

12.9 Summary

Task-specific training refers to training that uses gait itself to improve gait. For training individuals with severe impairments, external supports may be needed, such as robots, body weight support systems, and assistance from other healthcare providers. Expensive equipment may also be required, and such training can place a physical burden on both people with gait disabilities and healthcare providers. Moreover, task-specific training's superiority over other gait training methods remains unclear.

References

Calafiore D, Negrini F, Tottoli N, Ferraro F, Ozyemisci-Taskiran O, de Sire A. Efficacy of robotic exoskeleton for gait rehabilitation in patients with subacute stroke: a systematic review. Eur J Phys Rehabil Med. 2022;58(1):1–8.

Duncan PW, Sullivan KJ, Behrman AL, Azen SP, Wu SS, Nadeau SE, Dobkin BH, Rose DK, Tilson JK, Cen S, Hayden SK, LEAPS Investigative Team. Body-weight-supported treadmill rehabilitation after stroke. N Engl J Med. 2011;364(21):2026–36.

Helbostad JL. Treadmill training and/or body weight support may not improve walking ability following stroke. Aust J Physiother. 2003;49(4):278.

Nedergård H, Arumugam A, Sandlund M, Bråndal A, Häger CK. Effect of robotic-assisted gait training on objective biomechanical measures of gait in persons post-stroke: a systematic review and meta-analysis. J Neuroeng Rehabil. 2021;18(1):64.

Pereira S, Mehta S, McIntyre A, Lobo L, Teasell RW. Functional electrical stimulation for improving gait in persons with chronic stroke. Top Stroke Rehabil. 2012;19(6):491–8.

Shumway-Cook A, Woollacott MH, Rachwani J, Santamaria V. Abnormal postural control (Chapter 10). In: Motor control: translating research into clinical practice. 6th ed. Philadelphia: Lippincott Williams & Wilkins; 2023. p. 247–80.

Stephenson JL, Lamontagne A, De Serres SJ. The coordination of upper and lower limb movements during gait in healthy and stroke individuals. Gait Posture. 2009;29(1):11–6.

13 Task-Oriented Gait Training

13.1 Definition of Task-Oriented Gait Training

Task-oriented gait training and task-specific gait training are terms that are sometimes used interchangeably, but they can be distinguished by their more specific scopes. Task-oriented gait training focuses on improving the performance of functional tasks and includes training aimed at reducing underlying impairments, part practice, and whole practice (Shumway-Cook et al. 2023). Whole task practice involves actual gait training, including overground walking, body weight-supported treadmill training (BWSTT), and robot training. It can also be referred to as task-specific gait training. Therefore, the range of task-oriented gait training is broad and includes task-specific gait training.

13.2 Evidence of Effectiveness of Task-Oriented Gait Training

Gait training is an essential component of rehabilitation, and its effectiveness is well established. There is substantial research providing evidence of the effectiveness of task-oriented gait training (Allin et al. 2020; Bhatt et al. 2012). For instance, a multidimensional exercise program significantly improved balance and Dynamic Gait Index (DGI) in older adults (≥75 years of age) (Shumway-Cook et al. 1997). A task-oriented approach also delivered intensive massed practice and was found to have improved balance in stroke patients (Vearrier et al. 2005; Duncan et al. 1998). Moreover, task-oriented training has been recommended by many guidelines (Diermayr et al. 2020).

13.3 Principles of Task-Oriented Gait Training

13.3.1 Strengthening Before Balance Training

Muscle strengthening and motor control training should be conducted before commencing standing balance training. If standing balance training is performed without adequate muscle strength and motor control, individuals may rely on compensatory strategies to complete tasks, potentially leading to an abnormal gait.

13.3.2 Maximize Function of the Affected Limb

It is essential to create a training plan that aims to maximize the function of the affected limb. To achieve this, forced use of the affected lower limb is necessary.

Y.-S. Lee, *Task Oriented Gait Training*, https://doi.org/10.1007/978-981-97-3348-4_13

13.3.3 Safety

Safety is the primary concern in gait training, encompassing not only safety during training sessions but also safety outside of treatment hours.

13.3.4 Progressive Training

Training should progress from easier tasks to more challenging ones as the function of people with gait disabilities improves.

13.4 Sequence of Gait Training

13.4.1 Muscle Strengthening of Weight-Supporting Muscles

The muscle strengthening method for people with upper motor neuron lesions is different from the muscle strengthening method for people with lower motor neuron lesions. If there is weakness due to lower motor neuron lesions, such as muscle weakness that occurs in elderly people, strengthening of the knee extensor and hip extensor is performed first. This is because hip and knee extensor muscles are essential for body weight support in a standing posture. After this is complete, muscle strengthening for the ankle plantar flexor muscles and the hip abductors is conducted. These muscles are essential for standing balance.

In the case of upper motor neuron lesions, the method varies depending on whether there is voluntary movement or not. Functional electrical stimulation, weight-bearing, and passive movement of the affected lower extremities are used to restore muscle strength when there is no voluntary movement in the affected lower extremity, such as in the case of hemiplegia due to a stroke. The sliding tilt table is useful for people with hemiplegia for training to restore muscle strength because it can provide passive motion to the affected lower extremity while the weight is loaded on the affected lower extremity. When people with hemiplegia train using a sliding tilt table, both knees should be tied with a band to control the external rotation of the affected hip joint because the hip internal rotator lacks the muscle strength to control the external rotation of the affected hip joint. If the voluntary movement of the hip internal rotator is restored even if it is weak, the muscle strengthening exercise for the hip internal rotator should be performed first. If the hip internal rotator is weak, strengthening of the hip flexor muscles or the extensor muscles of the lower extremity is done while the hip joint is externally rotated. If muscle strengthening continues while the hip joint is externally rotated, this movement becomes a habit, making it difficult to correct later. When training to strengthen the hip flexor or extensor muscles of the lower extremity, training should be done with control of the external rotation of the hip joint using contraction of the hip internal rotator. After the strength of the hip internal rotator muscle recovers to some extent, it is important to strengthen the hip and knee extensor muscles. This is because hip and knee extensor muscles are essential for body weight support in a standing posture. If the muscle strength of the hip and knee extensor muscles recovers to the extent that they can support the subject's body weight, balance training can be performed in a standing position. If there is a problem with sitting balance, sitting balance training is to be conducted at this time.

13.4.2 Training for Steady-State Standing Balance

Steady-state standing balance training can begin with the individual standing while placing a hand on the wall for support. As those with gait disabilities become more comfortable with standing, encourage them to shift their body weight toward their heels and reduce their reliance on the wall. Once they can maintain a standing position without placing their hands on the wall, they should practice standing without the use of their hand, gradually increasing the duration of their standing position. During steady-state standing balance training, it is essential to focus on strengthening the ankle plantar flexor muscles and hip abductors. When individuals can stand without touching the wall for over 30 seconds, they can progress to proactive balance training.

13.4.3 Training for Proactive Standing Balance

Proactive standing balance training starts with shifting the center of body mass forward and backward, as well as side to side, on level ground. Once individuals can perform these movements comfortably, they can move on to step-up exercises. During step-up training, the affected foot is placed on a step, and the unaffected foot is lifted from the floor and placed on the step using the force of the affected leg.

In the initial stages of step-up training, individuals can use their hands for balance by placing them against a wall. However, they should gradually reduce hand usage, so that eventually training can be conducted without hand usage. If step-up exercises are too challenging or unsafe, individuals can practice weight shifts or partial step-ups with the affected foot on the step.

Once step-up exercises are mastered, individuals can progress to step-down training. Initially, they can place their hands on the wall for balance, but they should progress toward performing step-downs without hand usage. Throughout proactive standing balance training, it is crucial to continue strengthening the ankle plantar flexor muscles and hip abductors.

The final steps in proactive standing balance training include step-down touches, foot reaches, and single-leg squats. These exercises involve similar joint movements in the supporting limb. Single-leg squat training can be done in narrow spaces to minimize the risk of falls, making it suitable for independent home training. Eventually, training can progress to overground gait training. A visual illustration of this sequence can help individuals more clearly understand the progression (Fig. 13.1).

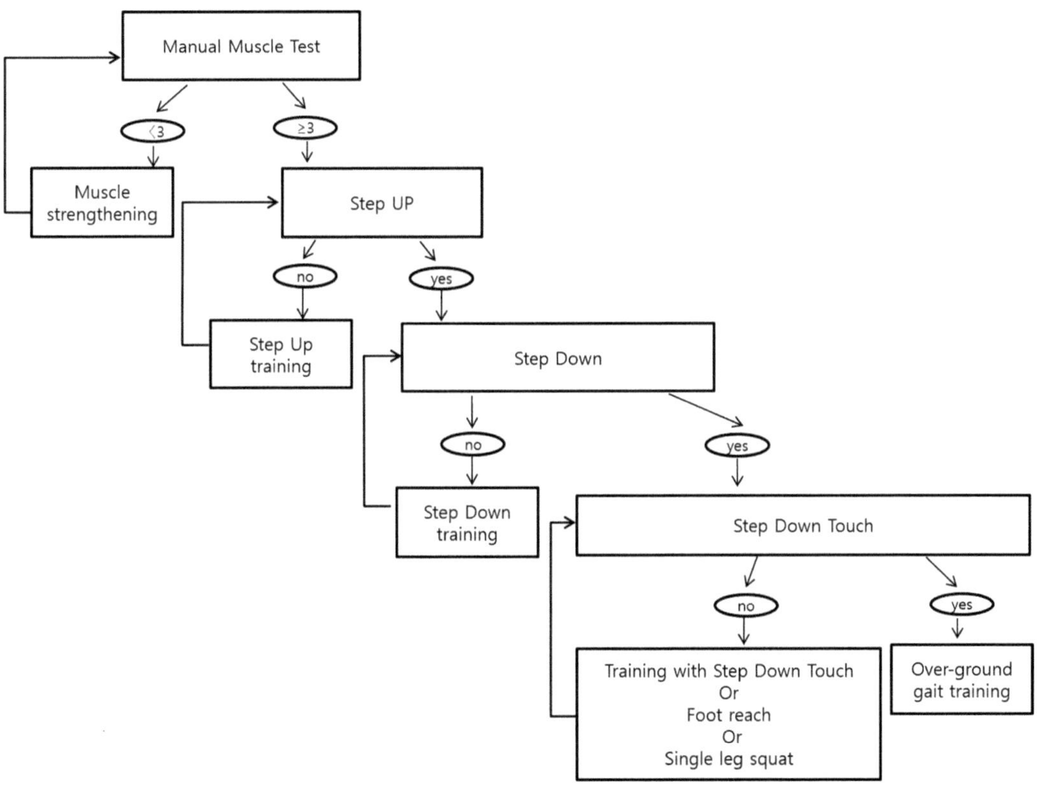

Fig. 13.1 Flow diagram of step-by-step task-oriented gait training. After muscle strengthening, training can advance to step-ups, step-downs, and step-down touches (or foot reaches and single-leg squats). Note that many details were omitted to keep the diagram from becoming too complicated

13.4.4 The Reasons for Placing Overground Gait Training at the End

Although overground gait training is easier than step-ups, the reasons for placing overground gait training at the end are as follows.

First, it minimizes the risk of falling. The risk of falls follows an inverted U shape (Homann et al. 2013). If people with gait disabilities start overground gait training without adequate balance, the risk of falling is high. Tasks like step-ups, step-downs, and step-down touches are in-place training exercises. When these tasks are performed near a wall, facing the wall, in narrow spaces, or with assistance from others, the risk of falling is minimal. By delaying overground gait training until people have regained adequate balance, it may be possible to minimize the risk of falling.

Second, it prevents abnormal gait. For example, if overground gait training starts before regaining adequate knee control, people with gait disabilities may become dependent on compensation strategies, potentially leading to an abnormal gait like genu recurvatum. If overground gait training begins after regaining adequate knee control, people with gait disabilities will not rely on compensation strategies, which can prevent an abnormal gait.

Third, it maximizes the gait function of people with gait disabilities. If people with gait disabilities start overground gait training before undergoing adequate training, many of them may resist more challenging training. They might be satisfied with achieving independent gait, even if it is not yet normal. In such cases, patients may fail to regain normal gait or maximize their gait function.

Fourth, it reduces the time needed for overground gait training. If people sufficiently regain the ability to control the joints of the affected limb, the time required for training in overground gait is significantly reduced or may not even be necessary.

13.4.5 Training People with Severe Ankle Plantar Flexor Weakness

Severe ankle plantar flexors make step-down-touch and single-leg squats impossible. Sometimes, recovery of ankle plantar flexor strength requires a long time. In such a case, overground gait training can be started after mastering the step-down. After regaining ankle plantar flexor muscle strength, training with the step-down-touch or single-leg squat can be started.

13.5 Advantages of Step-by-Step Task-Oriented Gait Training

First, this training can maximize the function of the affected limb and enhance gait function. By focusing on the forced use of the affected limb, it can maximize the function of the affected limb and improve overall gait function. Through this training, it may be possible for individuals with gait disabilities not only to walk on level ground but also to navigate stairs, slopes, and irregular terrain.

Second, this training can prevent abnormal gait patterns. By emphasizing the maximization of the affected limb's function and the avoidance of compensatory strategies, this training can effectively prevent abnormal gait patterns that may result from compensatory strategies.

Third, this training is easy to learn and perform. Its simplicity and ease of understanding make it easy to learn. Training in a standing position commences after individuals with gait disabilities have regained sufficient muscle strength in the affected lower limb, making it easy to perform. From the perspective of healthcare providers, the physical burden is minimal because they do not need to support the body weight of individuals with gait disabilities. From the perspective of people with gait disabilities, this training is very straightforward and comfortable in its execution because it progresses step by step in accordance with their functional improvement.

Fourth, this training does not require expensive equipment, such as body weight support systems, treadmills, or gait-training robots. Therefore, it can be implemented in any location worldwide.

13.6 Summary

Task-oriented gait training focuses on improving the performance of functional tasks and includes training aimed at reducing underlying impairments, part practice, and whole practice.

Step-by-step task-oriented gait training follows a systematic progression, starting with muscle strengthening and advancing through step-ups, step-downs, step-down touches (or foot reaches and single-leg squats), and concluding with overground gait training.

Step-by-step task-oriented gait training has many advantages, including the potential to maximize gait function and prevent abnormal gait patterns. It is also simple to learn and execute, while also being cost-effective as it does not require expensive equipment.

References

Allin LJ, Brolinson PG, Beach BM, Kim S, Nussbaum MA, Roberto KA, Madigan ML. Perturbation-based balance training targeting both slip- and trip-induced falls among older adults: a randomized controlled trial. BMC Geriatr. 2020;20:205.

Bhatt T, Yang F, Pai YC. Learning to resist gait-slip falls: long-term retention in community-dwelling older adults. Arch Phys Med Rehabil. 2012;93(4):557–64.

Diermayr G, Schomberg M, Greisberger A, Elsner B, Gronwald M, Salbach NM. Task-oriented circuit training for mobility in outpatient stroke rehabilitation in Germany and Austria: a contextual transferability analysis. Phys Ther. 2020;100(8):1307–22.

Duncan P, Richards L, Wallace D, Stoker-Yates J, Pohl P, Luchies C, Ogle A, Studenski S. A randomized, controlled pilot study of a home-based exercise program for individuals with mild and moderate stroke. Stroke. 1998;29(10):2055–60.

Homann B, Plaschg A, Grundner M, Haubenhofer A, Griedl T, Ivanic G, Hofer E, Fazekas F, Homann CN. The impact of neurological disorders on the risk for falls in the community dwelling elderly: a case-controlled study. BMJ Open. 2013;3(11):e003367.

Shumway-Cook A, Gruber W, Baldwin M, Liao S. The effect of multidimensional exercises on balance, mobility, and fall risk in community-dwelling older adults. Phys Ther. 1997;77(1):46–57.

Shumway-Cook A, Woollacott MH, Rachwani J, Santamaria V. Clinical management of the patient with a mobility disorder (Chapter 16). In: Motor control: translating research into clinical practice. 6th ed. Philadelphia: Lippincott Williams & Wilkins; 2023. p. 440–89.

Vearrier LA, Langan J, Shumway-Cook A, Woollacott M. An intensive massed practice approach to retraining balance post-stroke. Gait Posture. 2005;22(2):154–63.

Gait Training for People with Specific Diseases

14

14.1 Stroke

The most common walking disorders in people with stroke are hemiplegic gait and ataxic gait. Hemiplegic gait may result from learned nonuse and compensatory strategies. Step-by-step, task-oriented gait training, and restoration of motor function and balance before starting gait training in a standing posture may help prevent abnormal gait patterns. In most people with stroke, proximal muscles recover earlier than distal muscles.

Initially, sitting balance training and the strengthening of proximal muscles, including the hip internal rotators, are performed. If hip flexor and knee extensor strengthening begins without adequate strength of the hip internal rotators, individuals with stroke may have difficulty controlling hip external rotation. This can become a habitual movement pattern, in which hip flexion and knee extension are accompanied by hip external rotation. Excessive hip external rotation during gait is not only visually unusual but also impairs weight-bearing on the affected lower limb.

After regaining strength in the hip internal rotators, it is possible to start strengthening the hip extensors and knee extensors. If individuals with stroke achieve adequate muscle strength to support their body weight using only the affected lower limb, balance training in a standing position can be initiated. Step-by-step balance training can include steady-state standing, step-ups, step-downs, and step-down touches (or foot reaches and single-leg squats) in that order.

If possible, it is recommended that subjects commence walking training after regaining sufficient balance. Through this training, individuals with stroke can achieve maximal recovery of gait function. People with pure ataxic gait typically have enough muscle strength. Therefore, only balance training and overground gait training, as mentioned above, are required.

Some people with stroke may experience anosognosia and overestimate their balance and gait function. In such cases, it may be helpful to simulate a fall while using an overhead harness for safety. Through this experience, individuals with anosognosia may recognize their disability.

14.2 Traumatic Brain Injury

In many aspects, gait abnormalities in people with traumatic brain injury are similar to those observed in people with stroke. However, many individuals with traumatic brain injury experience decreased alertness. Transitioning them into a sitting position may help improve alertness. Since people with impaired alertness may be unable to report symptoms of orthostatic hypotension, moving them to a sitting position should only be done after confirming the absence of orthostatic hypotension.

Y.-S. Lee, *Task Oriented Gait Training*, https://doi.org/10.1007/978-981-97-3348-4_14

14.3 Spinal Cord Injury

In people with incomplete spinal cord injuries, the goal of gait training should be to achieve normal or near-normal gait because there is a possibility of regaining normal gait. Many individuals with incomplete spinal cord injuries have symmetric motor and sensory impairments. In such cases, strengthening can be done with both lower extremities simultaneously. However, balance training should be carried out one leg at a time as regaining normal gait requires the patient to support themselves and maintain balance with one lower limb only. Controlling the center of mass during single-leg support in the gait cycle is the most challenging aspect of gait.

To regain normal gait, individuals should focus on tasks that primarily use one leg, such as step-ups, step-downs, and step-down touches (or foot reaches, and single-leg squats), in that order. Although people with incomplete spinal cord injuries may not fully regain walking function, regaining the ability to support their body weight using two affected lower limbs can be extremely helpful. In such cases, individuals with spinal cord injuries can stand by themselves, which is beneficial for activities like transferring from a bed to a wheelchair and assuming a standing posture.

In contrast, for people with complete spinal cord injuries, regaining walking function is very challenging. While individuals with complete paraplegia can walk using crutches and knee-ankle-foot orthoses, this method is not functional due to its excessive energy consumption. They may choose wheelchair ambulation as their primary mode of locomotion, especially if they lack adequate hip flexion strength. Healthcare providers should consider this situation when setting goals and designing training programs. It is advisable to have a discussion with individuals who have spinal cord injuries about the long-term outcomes and options.

There are many robot systems designed to assist in regaining gait function, but they are often impractical due to their high cost, the inconveniences of wearing and removing them, the need for lengthy training, and the required cardiopulmonary function.

Wheelchairs remain a practical option for individuals with complete spinal cord injuries. However, recent advancements in technology, such as brain–computer interfaces, digital bridges, and epidural electrical stimulation, offer promising possibilities for enabling independent walking in people with complete spinal cord injuries (Lorach et al. 2023).

14.4 Parkinson's Disease

Many people with Parkinson's disease experience gait disabilities. Representative features of abnormal gait in individuals with Parkinson's disease include limited hip and knee extension, a forward-leaning trunk, and short step lengths. These individuals often exhibit slow walking velocity, shorter and more variable step lengths, longer stride durations, increased stance periods (mainly double support time), and a corresponding decrease in the swing phase of their gait.

During the stance period, observations include the loss of heel strike, incomplete knee extension during mid-stance, and loss of plantar flexion of the ankle in terminal stance. Forward trunk lean, reduced trunk motion, and diminished arm swing can be observed in the entire gait cycle.

In the swing phase, a reduced amplitude and speed of lower limb motion, as well as diminished toe clearance, are observed. These gait changes can also occur in healthy individuals walking on slippery surfaces, suggesting that balance problems may contribute to these alterations in gait patterns in people with Parkinson's disease.

Freezing of gait is a common occurrence in people with late-stage Parkinson's disease, appearing as decreased or loss of foot movement during gait initiation, turning, passing through narrow doorways, reaching a destination, or while performing secondary tasks (Snijders et al. 2007). While various approaches, including medications, surgeries, physiotherapy, and walking aids, are currently used to address freezing of gait, it remains a challenging hurdle (Nonnekes et al. 2015). Since these situations require more cognitive resources, they are similar to dual-task performance. Thus, improving gait function and balance may reduce freezing of gait.

Festinating gait is another typical gait abnormality in people with Parkinson's disease or Parkinson's syndrome. In festinating gait, the walking velocity progressively increases, and stop becomes more difficult. This may be a compensatory strategy aimed at regaining balance.

Sometimes, individuals with advanced Parkinson's disease can respond quickly to environmental events and exhibit unexpected mobility (i.e., kinesia paradoxical). It appears that individuals with Parkinson's disease can use external triggers to engage alternative motor circuits and bypass the defective basal ganglia circuitry (Wu and Hallett 2005). Therefore, external cues are widely used to improve gait disability in patients with Parkinson's disease (Nonnekes et al. 2019).

Balance training can enhance balance in people with Parkinson's disease (Wong-Yu and Mak 2015; Conradsson et al. 2015). Consequently, improving balance through training may be a more beneficial strategy for addressing gait disabilities in individuals with Parkinson's disease. To improve balance, step-by-step balance training can be performed, including steady-state standing, step-ups, step-downs, and step-down touches (or foot reaches and single-leg squats), in that order.

14.5 Cerebral Palsy

Many people with cerebral palsy have spasticity, and spasticity may cause abnormal gait, such as a crouch gait or scissoring gait.

People with diplegia often have hamstring spasticity and adductor spasticity. The crouch-gait pattern is a result of hamstring spasticity. Hamstring spasticity causes a short step length, a slow walking speed, and an increased energy cost of gait.

Hip adductor spasticity leads to adduction of the lower limbs and may cause a scissoring gait, impeding forward movement of the swing limb. Hip adductor spasticity interferes with hip abduction, which is an important compensation mechanism for poor balance, thus affecting stability.

Many individuals with cerebral palsy walk less as they get older and increasingly rely on a wheelchair due to the increased energy cost of walking (Palisano et al. 2009). Increased body weight and size may also contribute to this increase in energy cost.

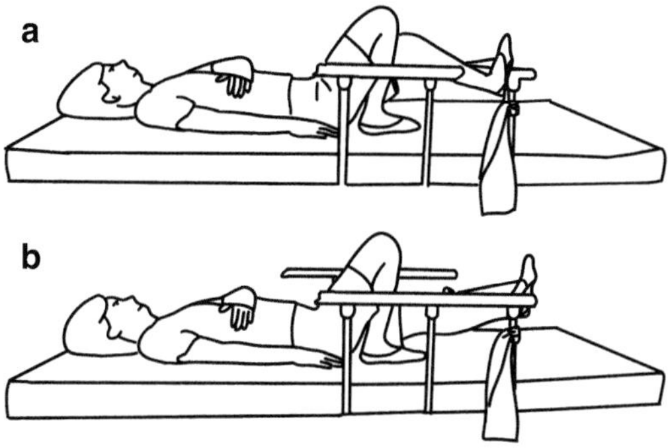

Fig. 14.1 Strengthening of antigravity muscles of lower extremity with rubber band. A rubber band fixed to the safety bars can be used to do strengthening training of extensor muscles of the lower extremity. (**a**) Starting position, (**b**) Final position

Maladaptive plasticity is one of the important causes of spasticity (Li et al. 2021). Therefore, step-by-step training may prevent spasticity in people with cerebral palsy.

Training can begin with sitting balance training and muscle strengthening. Muscle strengthening in a lying-down position using a rubber band (Fig. 14.1) or a sliding tilt table may increase the strength of body weight support muscles without aggravating spasticity.

Afterward, training can progress to the next stage, which is standing balance training. This can include steady-state standing, step-ups, step-downs, and step-down touches (or foot reaches and single-leg squats), in that order.

14.6 Knee Osteoarthritis

Many people with gait disabilities experience knee pain, and knee osteoarthritis is the main cause of knee pain.

People with knee pain often require pain control before training. Medication may be the first choice for pain control, but other methods such as strengthening and changing joint alignment are also important.

While strong muscles can protect the knee joint, sometimes muscle strengthening can actually provoke knee pain. Isotonic exercise is commonly used for muscle strengthening. People experience more pain when the joints are more flexed; therefore, the range of motion of the knee joint should be decreased.

Since knee pain can worsen with joint flexion, decreasing the degree of maximal joint flexion and increasing the inclination angle while training with a sliding tilt table can be helpful.

If people feel pain while exercising with a decreased range of motion, strengthening via isometric exercise may be helpful. Isometric exercise is used mainly because isotonic exercise may increase joint stress in people with arthritis. Because dynamic exercises with free weights or body weight may put stress on the joints, strengthening for people with osteoarthritis can be done through the use of a band (elastic or nonelastic) using isometric exercise in the supine position.

But isometric exercise is not interesting, so most people do not wish to continue exercising this way. The quadriceps-setting exercise is a well-known isometric exercise, but it is somewhat boring. However, exercise with an elastic band is often considered less boring than the quadriceps-setting exercise.

It is possible to perform exercise while maintaining full extension in the knee joints and while flexing the hip joint of one lower extremity and extending the hip joint of the other lower extremity with a rubber band on the ankles. In this training, each lower extremity moves in the opposite direction, like in a game of tug-of-war. After maintaining maximal muscle contraction for 5 s, change the direction of hip movement in the opposite direction. Ankle dorsiflexors can be contracted with hip flexion, and ankle plantar flexors can be contracted with hip extension simultaneously.

Figure 14.2 shows isometric knee strengthening exercise in the supine position with a rubber band.

It is possible to perform isometric exercises with weight-bearing in a standing position. Initially, stand with both legs, with the affected limb placed anteriorly. Shift body weight to the affected lower limb while maintaining partial knee flexion. It is possible to measure the amount of weight-bearing using a body weight scale.

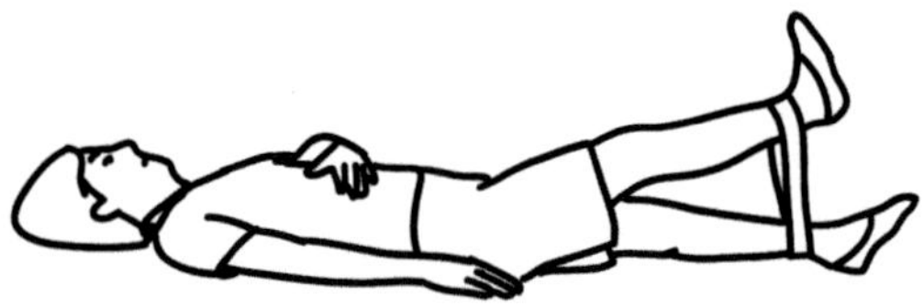

Fig. 14.2 Isometric strengthening exercise of the knee extensors with a rubber band

Changing the knee alignment and shifting the weight to the lateral portion of the knee joint may decrease knee pain. To control knee pain by altering the alignment of the knee joint in the coronal plane, high tibial osteotomy is widely performed (Lee and Byun 2012). People can also shift weight-bearing from the medial part of the knee joint to the lateral part of the knee joint by other means. In genu valgus, there is more weight-bearing on the lateral part of the knee joint than on the medial part. Shifting weight to the lateral portion of the knee joint is possible by bearing more weight on the medial side of the foot while performing tasks such as step-ups, step-downs, and step-down touches.

To shift weight to the medial part of the foot, contraction of the hip internal rotators and hip adductors is needed. If these muscles are weak, strengthening them is necessary.

14.6.1 Hip Surgery

As the aging population grows in size, the number of hip surgeries, including total hip replacement, is increasing. Hip replacement surgery might be an option if hip pain interferes with daily activities and other surgical procedures have not helped or are no longer effective. Hip fractures and arthritis damage are the common reasons for hip replacement.

Many people use a cane after total hip surgery even if they did not use one before the surgery. People who have a risk of decreased walking ability need rehabilitation training, and this is especially true for elderly individuals and those with comorbidities.

Initially, strengthening the muscles around the hip joint is necessary. Training with a sliding tilt table is very useful for strengthening the body weight support muscles. Through this method, it is possible to exercise in a lying-down position while also being easy to adjust the resistance. With a sliding tilt table, people with hip surgery can experience weight-bearing with the affected lower limb.

Gait training after total hip surgery can be done at home using an elastic band, a body weight scale, and a safety bar. Training with an elastic band is also very useful as it allows for the strengthening of not only the body weight support muscles but also other muscles around the hip, such as the hip adductors.

By placing the foot of the hip that was operated on a body weight scale and holding onto a safety bar, the people can train weight-bearing on the affected lower limb using feedback regarding the amount of weight-bearing.

Depending on the stability of the operation site, it is possible to increase weight-bearing on the affected lower limb with further training. If people can bear their full body weight on the affected lower limb, they can try lifting the heel of the unaffected lower extremity.

If people can lift the heel of the unaffected lower extremity without difficulty, they can try briefly lifting the entire foot. After this, they can gradually move on to increasing the time of foot lift.

After the people can lift the foot of the unaffected lower extremity without difficulty, training can progress to step-ups. To perform a step-up, lift the foot of the unaffected lower extremity and place it on the step.

Once the patient can perform step-ups without difficulty, training can progress to step-downs and step-down touches, in that order.

Through this progressive step-by-step, task-oriented gait training, people with hip surgery can maximize their walking ability.

14.7 Elderly People with Gait Disability

Gait disorders are common in elderly people, and their prevalence increases with age, ranging from 15% at the age of 60 to 82% at the age of 88 (Bloem et al. 1992; Sudarsky 2001). Many elderly individuals walk slowly, exhibiting a shuffling and cautious walking pattern, often referred to as senile gait disorder (Snijders et al. 2007). However, it is important to note that 18% of very old individuals walk normally, so senile gait disorder is not inevitable (Bloem et al. 1992).

Many elderly people experience balance problems, leading to cautious gait patterns characterized by slow movement, a wide base, short strides, minimal trunk movement, bent knees, and elbows (Snijders et al. 2007). Slow walking with short step length, low cadence, and reduced proportion of the swing period are common gait abnormalities in the elderly. Other abnormal gaits may also result in a slow walking speed but usually involve focal abnormalities like genu recurvatum, foot drop, or trunk leaning.

This change in gait is similar to that exhibited by individuals walking on slippery surfaces or in darkness (Shumway-Cook et al. 2023a). Cautious gait is common among the elderly and is often related to a fear of falling (Giladi et al. 2005). People with cautious gait can be classified into two groups: those with an excessive fear of falling, leading to actual instability, and those with an appropriate level of fear considering their degree of instability (Snijders et al. 2007).

While slow walking in elderly people may be considered a normal part of aging, it is better classified as abnormal gait for several reasons. First, although the causes of slow walking speed are diverse, ranging from muscle weakness to balance problems and poor cardiopulmonary function, it can often be improved with appropriate training. Second, the normal range of gait speed in elderly people is based on general populations, but data collected from healthy elderly individuals can closely resemble that of young people.

Older adults who walk with a cautious gait may have a high risk of losing balance in the medial-lateral direction (Yamaguchi and Masani 2019). Balance ability, leg muscle strength, the availability of sensory information, and cognitive factors all contribute to changes in gait patterns (Shumway-Cook et al. 2023b).

Gait changes in older adults are more related to the loss of balance control than to muscle weakness (Murray et al. 1969). Cautious gait may be a compensatory gait pattern aimed at increasing stability (Murray et al. 1969, 1970). Increased coactivation of agonist and antagonist muscles at a joint to increase joint stiffness may be used to improve balance control (Woollacott et al. 1998).

Muscle weakness is another major cause of abnormal gait in the elderly. Early signs of gait disability include a slow speed, an abnormal gait pattern, and a fear of falling. To screen for slow speed, a gait velocity less than 1 meter per second can be used.

As people age, they lose muscle strength and balance ability, leading many to consider using a cane due to the fear of falling. However, once people start using a cane, they may become dependent on it, making it difficult to walk without it. With training, elderly individuals can improve their muscle strength and balance capabilities, potentially eliminating the need for a cane.

Since cautious gait is often linked to balance problems, balance training may help improve it. There is evidence that balance training can enhance balance performance in healthy older adults (Lesinski et al. 2015; Alizadehsaravi et al. 2022).

Resistance training can also increase muscle strength in healthy older adults (Borde et al. 2015).

Step-by-step, task-oriented gait training may be helpful in improving gait function. If muscle strengthening is required, it should be completed before balance training. In elderly people, weakness is usually symmetric. As such, strengthening with body weight using both lower limbs can be very useful, such as through such movements as sit-to-stands, bridging, and heel lifts. If the weakness is not severe, strengthening using only one lower limb may be more helpful.

Once elderly individuals regain enough antigravity muscle strength, balance training can progress to exercises such as step-ups, step-downs, and step-down touches (or foot reaches and single-leg squats), in that order.

14.8 Summary

The most common walking disorder in people with stroke is hemiplegic gait. Hemiplegic gait may result from learned nonuse and compensatory strategies to impairment. Step-by-step, task-oriented gait training, restoration of motor function, and balance before starting gait training may help prevent abnormal gait patterns.

It is important to note that maladaptive neural plasticity may contribute to the development of spasticity, making step-by-step training a potential preventive measure.

Many people who have undergone hip surgery experience also gait disabilities. Proper gait training following hip surgery can help maximize their gait function and overall mobility.

Abnormal gait is common among elderly individuals, often stemming from problems related to balance loss and muscle weakness. Early detection and intervention are crucial because there is evidence that balance training and strengthening exercises can be effective in improving muscle strength and balance in the elderly.

References

Alizadehsaravi L, Bruijn SM, Muijres W, Koster RAJ, van Dieën JH. Improvement in gait stability in older adults after ten sessions of standing balance training. PLoS One. 2022;17(7):e0242115.

Bloem BR, Haan J, Lagaay AM, van Beek W, Wintzen AR, Roos RA. Investigation of gait in elderly subjects over 88 years of age. J Geriatr Psychiatry Neurol. 1992;5(2):78–84.

Borde R, Hortobágyi T, Granacher U. Dose-response relationships of resistance training in healthy old adults: a systematic review and meta-analysis. Sports Med. 2015;45(12):1693–720.

Conradsson D, Löfgren N, Nero H, Hagströmer M, Ståhle A, Lökk J, Franzén E. The effects of highly challenging balance training in elderly with Parkinson's disease: a randomized controlled trial. Neurorehabil Neural Repair. 2015;29(9):827–36.

Giladi N, Herman T, Reider-Groswasser II, Gurevich T, Hausdorff JM. Clinical characteristics of elderly patients with a cautious gait of unknown origin. J Neurol. 2005;252:300–6.

Lee DC, Byun SJ. High tibial osteotomy. Knee Surg Relat Res. 2012;24(2):61–9.

Lesinski M, Hortobágyi T, Muehlbauer T, Gollhofer A, Granacher U. Effects of balance training on balance performance in healthy older adults: a systematic review and meta-analysis. Sports Med. 2015;45(12):1721–38.

Li S, Francisco GE, Rymer WZ. A new definition of poststroke spasticity and the interference of spasticity with motor recovery from acute to chronic stages. Neurorehabil Neural Repair. 2021;35(7):601–10.

Lorach H, Galvez A, Spagnolo V, Martel F, Karakas S, et al. Walking naturally after spinal cord injury using a brain–spine interface. Nature. 2023;618:126–33.

Murray MP, Kory RC, Clarkson BH. Walking patterns in healthy old men. J Gerontol. 1969;24(2):169–78.

Murray MP, Kory RC, Sepic SB. Walking patterns of normal women. Arch Phys Med Rehabil. 1970;51(11):637–50.

Nonnekes J, Snijders AH, Nutt JG, Deuschl G, Giladi N, Bloem BR. Freezing of gait: a practical approach to management. Lancet Neurol. 2015;14(7):768–78.

Nonnekes J, Ružicka E, Nieuwboer A, Hallett M, Fasano A, Bloem BR. Compensation strategies for gait impairments in parkinson disease: a review. JAMA Neurol. 2019;76(6):718–25.

Palisano RJ, Kang LJ, Chiarello LA, Orlin M, Oeffinger D, Maggs J. Social and community participation of children and youth with cerebral palsy is associated with age and gross motor function classification. Phys Ther. 2009;89(12):1304–14.

Shumway-Cook A, Woollacott MH, Rachwani J, Santamaria V. Control of normal mobility (Chapter 12). In: Motor control: translating research into clinical practice. 6th ed. Philadelphia: Lippincott Williams & Wilkins; 2023a. p. 333–66.

Shumway-Cook A, Woollacott MH, Rachwani J, Santamaria V. Aging and mobility (Chapter 14). In: Motor control: translating research into clinical practice. 6th ed. Philadelphia: Lippincott Williams & Wilkins; 2023b. p. 389–406.

Snijders AH, van de Warrenburg BP, Giladi N, Bloem BR. Neurological gait disorders in elderly people: clinical approach and classification. Lancet Neurol. 2007;6(1):63–74.

Sudarsky L. Gait disorders: prevalence, morbidity, and etiology. Adv Neurol. 2001;87:111–7.

Wong-Yu IS, Mak MK. Multi-dimensional balance training programme improves balance and gait performance in people with Parkinson's disease: a pragmatic randomized controlled trial with 12-month follow-up. Parkinsonism Relat Disord. 2015;21(6):615–21.

Woollacott MH, Burtner P, Jensen J, Jasiewicz J, Roncesvalles N, Sveistrup H. Development of postural responses during standing in healthy children and children with spastic diplegia. Neurosci Biobehav Rev. 1998;22(4):583–9.

Wu T, Hallett M. A functional MRI study of automatic movements in patients with Parkinson's disease. Brain. 2005;128:2250–9.

Yamaguchi T, Masani K. Effects of age-related changes in step length and step width on the required coefficient of friction during straight walking. Gait Posture. 2019;69:195–201.

Abnormal Gait 15

15.1 Cautious Gait

Cautious gait refers to an abnormal gait due to a fear of falling. It usually occurs in elderly people but can also occur in younger individuals with other comorbidities. Considering the large aging population, cautious gait may be the most common gait abnormality.

This gait appears slow, with a wider base than normal, reduced arm swing, and a slightly stooped posture. Many people with cautious gait use a cane, but balance training may be a better strategy because it can improve balance and may eliminate the need for the use of a cane altogether (Lesinski et al. 2015). More detailed information about balance training is mentioned in the chapter on balance training in this book. If there is a difference between actual balance and perceived balance, it can be helpful to have the subject perform difficult tasks while using an overhead harness.

15.2 Genu Recurvatum (Knee Hyperextension)

Genu recurvatum refers to hyperextension of the knee joint during the stance period of gait. Continued walking with genu recurvatum may reinforce abnormal gait. To correct genu recurvatum, walking with genu recurvatum should be minimized or prohibited.

Genu recurvatum can be caused by various impairments, including spasticity of the quadriceps or ankle plantar flexors, contractures of the ankle joint or ankle plantar flexor muscles, weakness of the knee extensor and ankle plantar flexor, and poor control of the knee extensor. Finding the exact cause is the first step, and it can be determined through a physical examination.

Although some people have enough muscle strength in the knee extensor, poor control of the knee extensor can result in genu recurvatum. Eccentric control of the knee extensor is more challenging than concentric control in people with upper motor neuron lesions. Training of eccentric contraction can be effectively done in a lying-down position using a sliding tilt table.

15.3 Poor Foot Clearance

Poor foot clearance can lead to tripping, prompting compensation strategies such as steppage gait or circumduction gait to avoid tripping. These compensation strategies not only impact the appearance of gait but also increase the energy cost of gait.

Poor foot clearance can be caused not only by weakness in ankle dorsiflexors or ankle plantar flexion contractures but also by decreased hip flexion. Poor foot clearance due to decreased hip flexion can be corrected with a high step gait, which involves exaggerating hip flexion while walking. Initially, training can be done with a subject's hands resting on the wall (Shumway-Cook et al. 2023). Training that

Y.-S. Lee, *Task Oriented Gait Training*, https://doi.org/10.1007/978-981-97-3348-4_15

involves repeated placement of the affected foot on a high box may also be helpful. In cases of severe weakness of the hip flexors, muscle strengthening can be done in a supine position using an elastic band.

If the cause of poor foot clearance is weakness of the ankle dorsiflexor, the first step is strengthening the ankle dorsiflexor. Muscle strengthening can be achieved through exercises, electrical stimulation therapy (for those with lower motor neuron lesions), or functional electrical stimulation (for those with upper motor neuron lesions). Strengthening the hip flexor is easier than strengthening the ankle dorsiflexor. Since the ankle dorsiflexors are mainly innervated by the corticospinal tract, it is challenging to regain ankle dorsiflexor strength in people with severe corticospinal system damage.

If it is impossible to restore ankle dorsiflexor function, an ankle-foot orthosis (AFO) can be used (Fig. 15.1).

Although AFOs correct foot drop, they restrict motion in the talocrural and subtalar joints, causing discomfort and abnormal joint motion. This problem is most severe when using rigid AFOs.

High-top shoes can partially correct foot drop and are more convenient to use while also being cosmetically appealing. To use high-top shoes or soft-type AFOs, there should be little or no increase in muscle tone in the ankle plantar flexors. If there is severe spasticity, it may be difficult to use high-top shoes and soft AFOs.

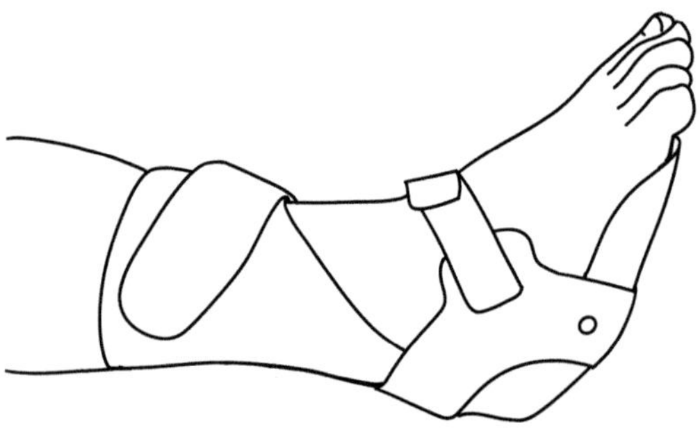

Fig. 15.1 Plastic ankle foot orthosis

15.4 Gait with Foot Inversion

Ankle inversion mainly occurs due to upper motor neuron lesions. It can lead to ankle inversion injuries, and some patients even experience ligament tears or malleolar fractures. Many patients also deal with worsening ankle inversion after prolonged walking. However, since continued walking with an abnormal gait pattern may exacerbate ankle inversion, it is helpful to correct foot inversion by stopping walking and instead training the people to adopt a normal gait. If correction through training is impossible, an AFO can correct ankle inversion. However, the use of an AFO may be inconvenient, and it can also cause abnormal body motion as it restricts joint motion around the ankle.

15.5 Circumduction Gait

Circumduction gait refers to an abnormal gait in which the leg moves in a semicircular pattern to advance the leg. It is used as a compensation method for poor hip flexion. Circumduction gait results in an unnatural gait pattern and increased energy expenditure, so it requires correction.

Correction can be achieved through the strengthening of hip flexor muscles. If the muscle strength of the hip flexors is very weak, such as with a strength level of grade 2, strengthening can be done in a supine position. Additionally, another person can assist the subject in strengthening the hip flexors. To do this, the hip joint and knee joint are first placed in partial flexion by another person. Then individuals with gait disabilities can actively flex the hip joint further by themselves.

People with weakness may find training in a supine position more comfortable than training in a side-lying position. It is also possible to strengthen the hip flexors without assistance from another person by using an elastic band. The elastic recoil of the stretched band can assist in hip flexor strengthening. The figure demonstrates the assistance of hip flexion contraction using an elastic band (Fig. 15.2).

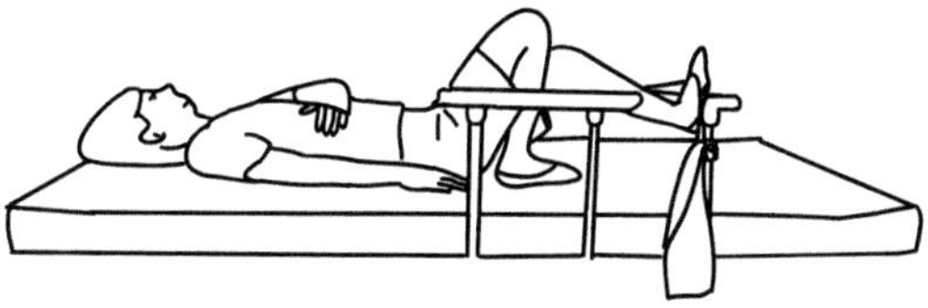

Fig. 15.2 Hip flexor strengthening using an elastic band

If the muscle strength of the hip flexors is at grade 3-, strengthening can be performed in a sitting position. If necessary, individuals can use their hands to provide a more stable sitting position by holding onto armrests or propping up on a mat with their hands. Muscle strength can be increased by performing hip flexion as high as possible. It is important to note that hip flexion in a sitting position is more challenging than in a supine position.

The next step is to strengthen the hip flexors in a standing position. Initially, strengthening can be done in a standing position with hands resting on the wall to help balance. Two methods can be used for strengthening: hip flexion in the air and stepping onto the top of a high box. With improvements in balance and strength, individuals can progress to training without using their hands for support.

15.6 Ataxic Gait

Ataxic gait refers to an abnormal gait caused by problems in cerebellar function. It is often characterized by reduced walking speed and cadence, reduced step length, stride length, and swing phase, increased step width, stride time, step time, and stance phase, and by a double-limb support phase, with increased variability of step length, stride length, and stride time (Buckley et al. 2018). Ataxic gait resembles the walking of a drunken person or walking performed on a rocking boat, characterized by a wide-based gait. It can be improved with balance training, and detailed information about balance training is provided in the chapter on balance training in this book.

15.7 Frontal Lobe Gait

Frontal lobe gait refers to a gait abnormality characterized by walking with short, shuffling steps and feet wide apart, while arm swing remains normal (Thompson 2012). Freezing of gait can also occur in frontal lobe gait. This gait abnormality is likely due to damage to the frontal cortex and its connections with subcortical structures, including the basal ganglia, cerebellum, and brainstem (Thompson 2012). Frontal lobe gait is frequently observed in people with dementia, microvascular white matter disorders, and normal pressure hydrocephalus.

The major problem in frontal lobe gait is a balance issue. At the very least, balance training can be helpful in managing the early stages of frontal lobe gait.

15.8 Summary

Considering the size of the aging population, cautious gait may be the most common gait abnormality, and balance training can be used to effectively address this problem.

Even when people have sufficient muscle strength in the knee extensors, poor control of these muscles can lead to genu recurvatum. Training in a lying down position, particularly using a sliding tilt table, is highly beneficial for improving knee control, specifically eccentric contraction.

Circumduction gait refers to an abnormal gait in which the leg moves in a semicircular pattern to advance the leg. It is used as a compensation for poor hip flexion. Correction of circumduction gait can be achieved through the strengthening of the hip flexor muscles.

References

Buckley E, Mazzà C, McNeill A. A systematic review of the gait characteristics associated with cerebellar ataxia. Gait Posture. 2018;60:154–63.

Lesinski M, Hortobágyi T, Muehlbauer T, Gollhofer A, Granacher U. Effects of balance training on balance performance in healthy older adults: a systematic review and meta-analysis. Sports Med. 2015;45(12):1721–38.

Shumway-Cook A, Woollacott MH, Rachwani J, Santamaria V. Clinical management of the patient with a mobility disorder (Chapter 16). In: Motor control: translating research into clinical practice. 6th ed. Philadelphia: Lippincott Williams & Wilkins; 2023. p. 440–89.

Thompson PD. Frontal lobe ataxia. Handb Clin Neurol. 2012;103:619–22.

16 Others

16.1 Other Gait Training

After regaining independent gait, other training can be conducted, including dual-task training, training with obstacles, adding additional movements during gait, changing the base of support, altering sensory input, and reactive balance training.

In daily life, various types of walking are utilized, such as walking backward or sideways and walking on a narrow base. Training with different walking directions may be helpful in improving gait function. The ability to negotiate curbs or obstacles is also necessary for community walking.

When people encounter an obstacle, they typically use two strategies: turning around or stepping over the obstacle. To train for stepping over obstacle, it is possible to use a light cone or a paper box (Fig. 16.1).

Light obstacles are possibly better than heavy ones because the risk of tripping is lower, and feedback can be enhanced. Progression can be made by increasing the size, number, width, and fragility of obstacles.

To improve gait function, sometimes additional movements can be incorporated during gait, such as turning one's head to locate an object or changing direction with a pivot turn.

In the real world, there are diverse bases of support. Gait training with various bases of support may be needed to prepare for a return to real-life situations. This may include soft surfaces (such as carpeted areas), hard surfaces, uneven ground, inclined surfaces, and narrow paths (Shumway-Cook et al. 2023b).

Balance training and gait training can be conducted by altering sensory input. Visual input can be changed by closing one's eyes, wearing sunglasses, or by using eyeglasses that are covered in petroleum gel. Vestibular input can be modified through head rotation and flexion, as well as by extension of the neck.

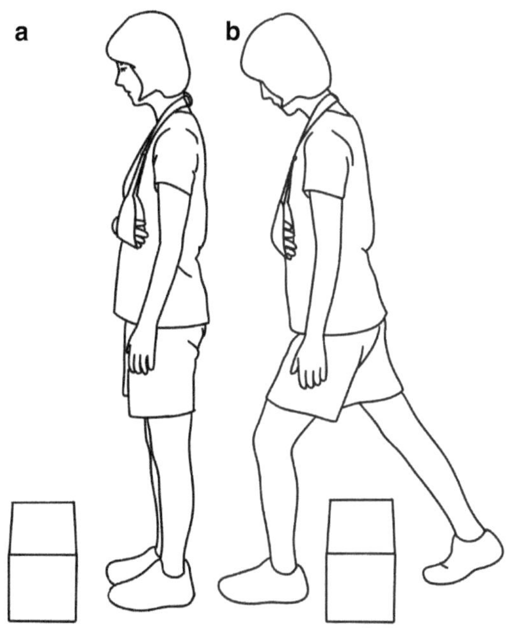

Fig. 16.1 Step over an obstacle. Practicing step over obstacle can help enable walking in a variety of situations. (**a**) Starting position, (**b**) Midpoint of step over an obstacle

Y.-S. Lee, *Task Oriented Gait Training*, https://doi.org/10.1007/978-981-97-3348-4_16

A virtual reality (VR) system can increase motivation for gait training and may be helpful in improving gait. Currently, VR is somewhat expensive and inconvenient, but it may become more affordable with technological advancements. These training methods can contribute to improve walking function.

16.2 Training Using Dual Tasks

After regaining independent gait, further training can be done with the use of dual-task gait training. Talking, carrying a bag, and negotiating traffic while walking down the street are common tasks performed in everyday life.

The risk of falling increases in people with an inability to flexibly allocate attention between cognitive tasks and walking performance (Siu et al. 2008). Balance confidence is independently associated with dual-task gait performance (Liu-Ambrose et al. 2009). In dual-task gait training, people often face more difficulty than in gait training without other tasks. This preparation is crucial for real-life situations, such as talking with friends, answering questions, and carrying items while walking.

Dual-task gait training can involve either cognitive tasks or motor tasks. Diverse cognitive activities can be used, such as spelling words forward or backward, naming words beginning with letters A to K, counting backward by threes, and identifying the opposite direction of a ball toss.

Various motor activities can also be employed, such as holding a basket, carrying a tray with an upright peg (Fig. 16.2), and handling objects.

More detailed information can be found in other references (Shumway-Cook et al. 2023b).

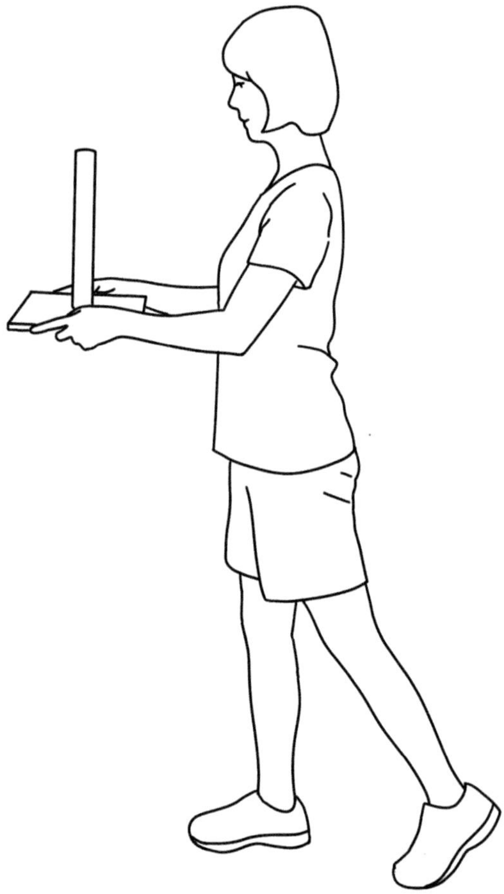

Fig. 16.2 Dual-task training that employs walking while carrying a tray containing an upright peg

16.3 Reactive Balance Training

Sometimes, people encounter perturbations due to unexpected external forces and must maintain balance using an appropriate response. Responses can be divided into in-place strategies and out-of-place strategies. In an in-place strategy, there is no change in the base of support after a perturbation. When using an out-of-place strategy, stepping or reaching for support with the upper extremities is utilized.

To induce perturbations, manual pushes or pulls, making people lean for support and then removing support, and abrupt changes in treadmill speed can be used (Shumway-Cook et al. 2023b). When performing these training activities, it is essential to use a gait belt or overhead harness in order to prevent falls (Shumway-Cook et al. 2023a).

16.4 Training Going Up and Down Stairs

After regaining overground gait, training to go up and down stairs may start. Going up and down stairs is associated with high musculoskeletal, balance, and cardiovascular demands, as well as a larger range of motion in the lower limb joints (Jacobs 2016; Startzell et al. 2000).

Going upstairs requires the generation of more concentric force at the knee for forward and vertical progression than is seen in overground walking (Shumway-Cook et al. 2023a). The forces needed for ascent are greater than those needed for walking on a level plane, with the knee extensors generating most of the energy required for stair ascent.

Since stair descent is achieved largely through eccentric contractions of the hip, knee, and ankle extensors, many people with upper motor neuron lesions (UMNL) have more difficulty with stair descent than with stair ascent. Knee extensors are the main source of the control of body weight during descent and present more hazardous conditions than in stair ascent (Tinetti et al. 1988).

Since the height of stairs (which are typically higher than 10 cm) is greater than that of a step (around 7.5 cm), starting stair training before mastering step-up and step-down can lead to learned nonuse of the affected lower limb and abnormal joint motion.

There are two strategies for using stairs: the compensatory strategy and the recovery strategy. In the compensatory strategy, the unaffected lower limb becomes the leading limb for stair ascent, and the affected lower limb becomes the leading limb for stair descent (Fig. 16.3).

While this strategy is easier for people with gait disabilities, it can lead to the learned misuse of the affected lower limb (Shumway-Cook et al. 2023b).

In the recovery strategy, the affected lower limb becomes the leading limb for stair ascent, and the unaffected lower limb becomes the leading limb for stair descent (Fig. 16.4).

Although this strategy is more challenging for people with gait disabilities, it can maximize the function and use of the affected lower limb.

Since the recovery strategy can maximize the function of the affected lower limb, it may be more beneficial than the compensatory strategy. However, as slow step-down movements require controlled flexion of the supporting lower limb, it is both more difficult and more effective for training purposes.

Sometimes, people with gait disabilities use handrails to compensate for weakness and poor balance. However, this can also result in the learned nonuse of the affected lower limb. During training,

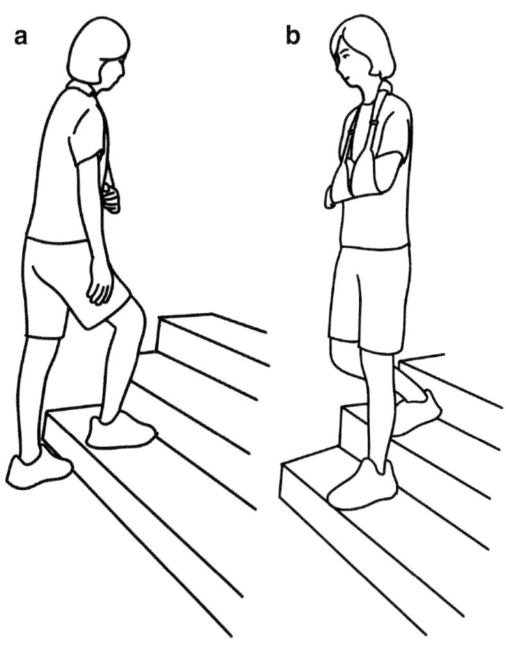

Fig. 16.3 Compensatory strategies: (**a**) stair ascent; (**b**) stair descent

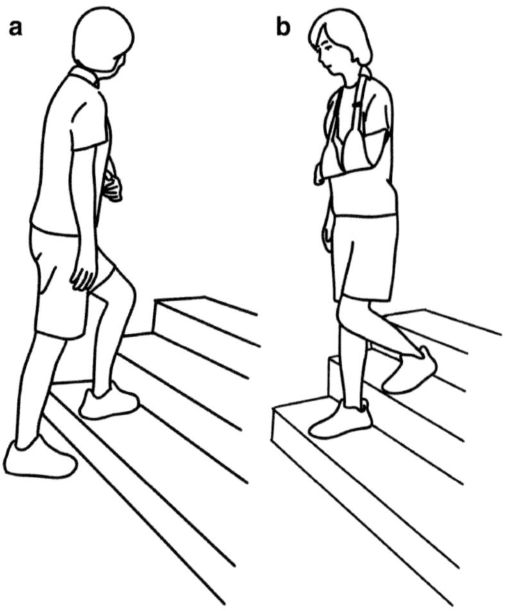

Fig. 16.4 Recovery strategies: (**a**) stair ascent; (**b**) stair descent

the use of hands should be minimized, and if possible, not using hands is better than using them.

16.5 Dizziness

Many people with gait disabilities experience dizziness, and the causes of dizziness are diverse. No matter the cause, though, it can have a significant impact on gait. One method to manage dizziness is habituation. People with dizziness can adapt to it through exposure to the movements that cause dizziness.

If head rotation to the right side causes dizziness, training should start with slow head rotation to right side, and with adaptation, the speed of rotation can be increased.

16.6 Sensory/Perception Test

16.6.1 Hemispatial Neglect

Hemispatial neglect can interfere with the detection of a dangerous environment and can lead to injury. Neglect can be tested while sitting, standing, or walking. Some people with neglect show hemispatial neglect only when walking. Therefore, testing for hemispatial neglect while walking may be necessary for individuals who have difficulty detecting dangers in their left visual field.

16.6.2 Proprioception

Proprioception can be tested by changing joint positions and moving body parts. When testing proprioception, holding the lateral side of the body is better because it makes it impossible for people to use their sense of pressure to compensate for the loss of proprioception.

Mirror movements by the contralateral limb can also be used in this test. To perform this test, the patient must catch the movement of the tested limb and mimic that movement accurately and rapidly using the contralateral limb.

Like other sensory systems, normal proprioception is extremely sensitive. As such, if a large movement arc is used, it may be impossible to detect slight or moderate sensory loss.

16.7 Program to Maintain Function

Gait training may be a lifelong process and can be divided into programs to both increase and maintain function. The effects of most gait training are temporary and fade over time. In other words, if training is stopped, the effects of gait training decay with time. Gait training for people with chronic stroke leads to small but significant improvements in mobility and gait speed, but these effects are not sustained without continued training (Green et al. 2002). The training effect on balance significantly decreases after step training (Rossi et al. 2013; Toulotte et al. 2006).

Since the training effect diminishes over time, a program aimed at maintaining function is absolutely essential. However, it is not practical to use the same training program for people with longstanding gait disabilities. The practical solution is to teach people with a gait disability how to perform gait training independently and then provide regular follow-up. The training should be easy to do and not require high expenses as it may be a lifelong process.

Strengthening can actually be performed with body weight or elastic bands, and balance training can be done with steps (e.g., with step-ups, step-downs, and step-down touches), single-leg squats, and foot reaches. Single-leg squats between a wall and a bed may be the best method of training at home. Aerobic exercise can be easily performed by walking. These exercises are simple and do not require expensive equipment.

If gait function deteriorates significantly, subjects may need supervised gait training or one-on-one gait training. Maintaining enough mobility to climb small hills may be a proper long-term goal. If people cannot climb small hills, they may require follow-up examinations by a medical practitioner. Although this approach requires some expenditure, it hugely reduces the societal cost while maintaining the quality of life of people with gait disabilities.

Because maintaining continued exercise is not easy, helpful methods are needed. Thus, it is necessary to prepare a program with the aim of maintaining function for people with residual gait disabilities after completing gait training. However, it is difficult to exercise for an extended period on one's own. As such, a strategy that can facilitate and help continuous exercise is needed.

One effective method is feedback. If people see the results of their training, it may be helpful. There are many simple tests used to assess training effects, such as the sit-to-stand test for lower extremity muscle strength and the 6-min walking test for endurance.

Secondly, recording and comparing past performance with present performance are valuable methods as well. Documenting training and comparing one's own function with that of others may be helpful. There are many apps that provide documentation and comparisons.

Third, exercising with appropriate equipment can make training easier to adhere to. Knee strengthening with leg presses or a sliding tilt table is easier than simply performing squat exercises.

Fourth, group exercise may be the most effective method of encouraging continued training. Exercising with friends and neighbors can make it a more enjoyable experience. As such, subjects may find it helpful to exercise with other people, such as family members, neighbors, or others with the same condition. Community-based programs that encourage social interactions in which people exercise together may help people maintain continuous exercise. Additionally, these programs may increase social participation (Nancy et al. 2015).

16.8 Walking Aids (Assistive Devices)

16.8.1 Cane

The reasons a person might use a cane are diverse, including weakness, poor balance, and pain. Many patients who use walking aids can increase muscle strength and balance through training, which can reduce their dependence on canes or even eliminate the need for them entirely. People who use canes are potential candidates for gait training. Canes provide additional sensory input, increase the base of support, and offer extra support against gravity (Shumway-Cook et al. 2023b). In the short term, it may decrease the incidence of falls. However, individuals may become psychologically dependent on canes and miss the opportunity to improve muscle strength and balance. Canes may also lead to asymmetry in gait and cause musculoskeletal problems in the upper extremities.

Therefore, canes should be provided only after appropriate training has demonstrated that there is no possibility of walking without a cane even after sufficient training. Without adequate training, people cannot achieve their maximal function, and there is a risk of learned nonuse of the affected body part. It is recommended to use the cane on the opposite side of the lesion, for people with femur problems, such as osteoarthritis, as this reduces compression force on the hip joint compared to using a cane on the same side.

There is no specific recommendation for which side is better in people with knee pathology. Using the cane on the unaffected side has two advantages: it increases the base of support during single-limb support of the affected limb and allows for a more normal arm swing because, typically, when one leg swings forward, the opposite arm swings forward. The ipsilateral arm and leg move reciprocally.

16.8.2 Stick

Sticks used in Nordic walking can improve stability and lead to faster gait speeds without an increased risk of falling in people with impaired balance. They may also help improve cardiopulmonary function.

16.8.3 Walker

Many people with acute illnesses restart walking with the use of a walker. However, the use of a walker may result in learned nonuse of the affected lower limb and interfere with the recovery of normal gait.

16.9 Orthoses

16.9.1 Ankle-Foot Orthoses

Ankle-foot orthoses are used to control foot inversion, foot drop, and genu recurvatum. They can also improve walking speed (Nascimento et al. 2020). However, ankle-foot orthoses has many limitations. They require time to put them on and take them off, may be unsightly due to the increased shoe size, and can block the normal motion of the tibiocrural joint and subtalar joint, potentially increasing energy costs and making walking more difficult.

Although there may be no voluntary motion in the ankle dorsiflexors, the ankle can be moved dorsally through associated movements in people with upper motor neuron lesions. Before prescribing an ankle-foot orthosis, actual gait should be observed. Many patients without ankle dorsiflexor strength may not need an ankle-foot orthosis. And if possible, high-top shoes may be a better solution than an ankle foot orthosis.

Genu recurvatum can be controlled with the use of an ankle-foot orthosis, but genu recurvatum may be used as compensation for the inability to control the knee. Knee control training may correct genu recurvatum. Therefore, checking knee control and providing training if needed should be done before prescribing an ankle-foot orthosis.

16.9.2 Knee Orthoses

Knee orthoses can be used to support knee extension. However, the use of a knee orthosis should be delayed because knee extensor strength can be increased through strengthening training, especially in cases of paresis due to brain lesions.

16.10 Summary

After regaining independent gait, additional training can be performed through the use of dual-task training, training with obstacles, incorporating other movements during gait, changing the base of support, altering sensory input, and reactive balance training.

Starting stair training before mastering the step-up and step-down may lead to learned nonuse of the affected lower limb and abnormal joint motion due to the greater height of stairs (which are typically higher than 10 cm) compared to steps (around 7.5 cm).

Since training effects diminish with time, a program aimed at maintaining function is absolutely necessary. Since gait training is a lifelong process, easy and cost-effective strategies are essential.

Many people who use walking aids can increase muscle strength and balance through training, reducing their dependency on canes or other walking aids.

Canes provide additional sensory input, increase the base of support, and offer extra support against gravity. In the short term, they may decrease the incidence of falls. However, individuals may become psychologically dependent on canes and miss the opportunity to improve muscle strength and balance.

References

Green J, Forster A, Bogle S, Young J. Physiotherapy for patients with mobility problems more than 1 year after stroke: a randomised controlled trial. Lancet. 2002;359:199–203.

Jacobs JV. A review of stairway falls and stair negotiation: lessons learned and future needs to reduce injury. Gait Posture. 2016;49:159–67.

Liu-Ambrose T, Katarynych LA, Ashe MC, Nagamatsu LS, Hsu CL. Dual-task gait performance among community-dwelling senior women: the role of balance confidence and executive functions. J Gerontol A Biol Sci Med Sci. 2009;64(9):975–82.

Nancy E, Mayo NE, Anderson S, Barclay R, Cameron JI, Desrosiers J, et al. Getting on with the rest of your life following stroke: a randomized trial of a complex intervention aimed at enhancing life participation post stroke. Clin Rehabil. 2015;29(12):1198–211.

Nascimento LR, da Silva LA, Barcellos JVMA, Teixeira-Salmela LF. Ankle-foot orthoses and continuous functional electrical stimulation improve walking speed after stroke: a systematic review and meta-analyses of randomized controlled trials. Physiotherapy. 2020;109:43–53.

Rossi LP, Pereira R, Brandalize M, Gomes ARS. The effects of a perturbation-based balance training on the reactive neuromuscular control in community-dwelling older women: a randomized controlled trial. Hum Mov. 2013;14(3):238–46.

Shumway-Cook A, Woollacott MH, Rachwani J, Santamaria V. Abnormal mobility. In: Motor control: translating research into clinical practice (Chapter 15). 6th ed. Philadelphia: Lippincott Williams & Wilkins; 2023a. p. 407–39.

Shumway-Cook A, Woollacott MH, Rachwani J, Santamaria V. Clinical management of the patient with a mobility disorder (Chapter 16). In: Motor control: translating research into clinical practice. 6th ed. Philadelphia: Lippincott Williams & Wilkins; 2023b. p. 440–89.

Siu KC, Chou LS, Mayr U, van Donkelaar P, Woollacott MH. Does inability to allocate attention contribute to balance constraints during gait in older adults? J Gerontol A Biol Sci Med Sci. 2008;63(12):1364–9.

Startzell JK, Owens DA, Mulfinger LM, Cavanagh PR. Stair negotiation in older people: a review. J Am Geriatr Soc. 2000;48(5):567–80.

Tinetti ME, Speechley M, Ginter SF. Risk factors for falls among elderly persons living in the community. N Engl J Med. 1988;319(26):1701–7.

Toulotte C, Thevenon A, Fabre C. Effects of training and detraining on the static and dynamic balance in elderly fallers and non-fallers: a pilot study. Disabil Rehabil. 2006;28(2):125–33.